FREEDOM FROM NEUROPATHY: FINDING LASTING RELIEF WITH L.E.G.A.C.Y.

Dr. Adam R. Tomasetti, DC
Freedom from Neuropathy: Finding Lasting Relief With
L.E.G.A.C.Y.

Published by Spines
ISBN: 979-8-89691-059-6

FREEDOM FROM NEUROPATHY: FINDING LASTING RELIEF WITH L.E.G.A.C.Y.

PROVEN METHODS TO OVERCOME MISERY AND ENJOY QUALITY OF LIFE

DR. ADAM R. TOMASETTI, DC

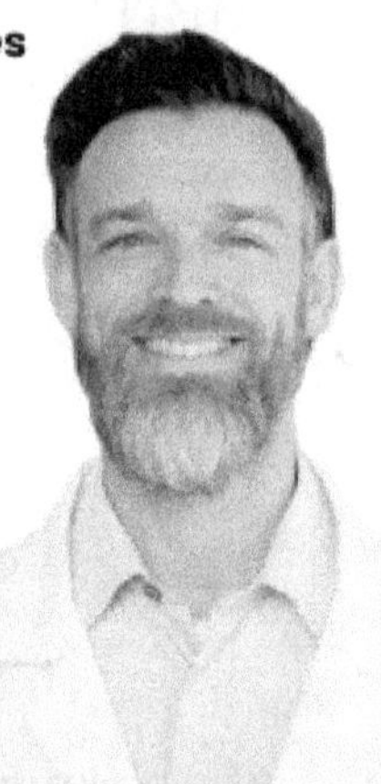

GET ACCESS TO YOUR
FREE REVERSING NEUROPATHY
GIFTS BELOW

LEGACYHEALTH

• Neuropathy Health Journal
• Reversing Neuropathy Guide
• 25 Anti-Inflammatory Recipes
• Nerve Damage Quiz
• Free Health Masterclass
• 30-Day Nutrition Plan
• Neuropathy Relief Handbook

SCAN ME DR. ADAM TOMASETTI DC

CONTENTS

FOREWORD

Neuropathy, a relentless thief of sensation and comfort, has long been a challenge for both patients and practitioners. It's a condition that can rob individuals of their quality of life, leaving them in a cycle of pain, numbness, and despair. But within these pages lies a beacon of hope, a testament to the power of innovation, and a roadmap towards reclaiming a life free from suffering.

Dr. Adam R. Tomasetti, D.C., with his extensive experience in chiropractic care and deep compassion for those who suffer from neuropathy, has poured his knowledge and unwavering dedication into creating a comprehensive guide that offers real solutions. *Freedom from Neuropathy: Finding Lasting Relief with L.E.G.A.C.Y.* is not merely a book; it is a lifeline, a testament to the transformative potential of the L.E.G.A.C.Y. Neuropathy Program.

As a fellow practitioner and Driven Doc member at The Data Driven Practice, I've had the privilege of witnessing firsthand the impact of Dr. Tomasetti's innovative approach. His unwavering commitment to patient care, his relentless pursuit of cutting-edge solutions, and his genuine empathy have touched countless lives.

In this book, Dr. Tomasetti generously shares his wealth of knowledge and experience, demystifying the complexities of neuropathy and empowering readers to take control of their health. The L.E.G.A.C.Y. Neuropathy Program, meticulously developed and refined through years of clinical practice, offers a holistic and evidence-based approach to not only managing but reversing neuropathy symptoms.

But *Freedom from Neuropathy: Finding Lasting Relief with L.E.G.A.C.Y.* is more than a collection of protocols. It's a testament to the resilience of the human spirit, a reminder that even in the face of adversity, there is always a path to healing.

With unwavering optimism and steadfast support, Dr. Tomasetti and his dedicated team at Legacy Health stand ready to guide you on your journey toward a misery-free life. This book is your first step, and I encourage you to embrace the wisdom within its pages. Your path to a brighter future starts here.

Sincerely,

Dr. Cory Frogley, D.C.
The Data Driven Practice

DISCLAIMER

Disclaimer: The information provided in this book is intended for educational purposes only and is not a substitute for professional medical advice. The author and publisher are not liable for any adverse effects or consequences resulting from the use of the information presented herein. Always consult your physician or a qualified healthcare provider regarding any health concerns or before making any decisions related to your health or treatment.

ABOUT THE AUTHOR

Hi, I'm Dr. Adam R. Tomasetti, D.C., an Applied Kinesiologist, Chiropractor, author, and I've spent years focused on understanding and treating neuropathy. My mission is simple: I want to help people overcome health challenges and live vibrant, pain-free lives. As the founder of L.E.G.A.C.Y, a breakthrough system that has helped many people find relief from neuropathy, I'm dedicated to sharing my knowledge and experience.

My journey with neuropathy wasn't something I planned – it became a personal mission driven by a profound experience. About a decade ago, my father had an accident triggered by the lasting neurological effects of his exposure to Agent Orange in Vietnam. The resulting fall left him paralyzed, permanently bound to a wheelchair- unable to fully hug his kids and grandkids again. LIving through the devastating impact on my father and our family drove me to find a way to prevent others from enduring the same heartbreak. I immersed myself in research, traveled the country, and sought out the world's leading neuropathy specialists.

My own challenges with chronic health issues as a teenager ignited my belief in natural healing. I had developed a persistent cough that lingered over 6 months. I couldn't speak 10 words without coughing. It defied conventional medicine- all the tests were normal. A skilled chiropractor highly trained in Applied Kinesiology who delved into the power of nutrition, stress reduction, and body alignment allowed me to completely resolve it within 2 weeks. Later, a car accident that numbed my left arm was corrected through a chiropractor specializing in functional neurology. Even my wife found freedom from debilitating GERD, ulcers and food allergies, thanks to the same Applied Kinesiology Doctor who treated me.

These experiences solidified my path. I pursued my doctorate in chiropractic with honors, became certified in Applied Kinesiology through the International College, and earned numerous advanced certifications, including the highest level III certification in Neuro Emotional Technique®. (I'll describe these techniques in more detail later). Each step was taken with the unwavering goal of mastering the intricate interplay of structure, chemistry and emotion in the human body . I then applied this backbone of knowledge and experience to the treatment of peripheral neuropathy. My years of focused study and practice culminated in the development of the L.E.G.A.C.Y. system – a unique and powerful approach rooted firmly in Applied Kinesiology and standard diagnostic testing to help determine which cutting-edge therapies and technologies to use and when to employ them- including Laser therapy, Pulsed Electromagnetic Field Therapy, nutrition, stress relief, detoxification, Allergy detection and elimination, Electromagnetic Stress modulation, nerve rehab and others.

I penned my book, "Freedom from Neuropathy: Finding Lasting Relief with L.E.G.A.C.Y.," to open a door to hope and healing. Within it, I chronicle my own journey, practical solutions, and the proven methods of my system – all offered in a way that's clear and empowering.

Today, I'm blessed to live in Camp Hill, Pennsylvania, with my wife and six children. Beyond my work, I treasure my relationship with God, my family time, reading, writing, and playing drums and some occasional ice hockey. Above all, my deepest passion remains the same: helping people to experience and enjoy all that God has for them in their life.

Please enjoy reading my book – and know that a better life is within your reach.

1

———

THE HIDDEN EPIDEMIC: NEUROPATHY'S IMPACT ON LIVES

When I first met Elvin, He could barely look me in the eye. I could tell he was worried. He'd lost a lot; his livelihood as a contractor, his social life was extremely limited, and worst of all, he'd lost hope. He was told by a neurologist that "there was nothing that could be done" for his neuropathy and that he would someday be crippled, losing his ability to walk on his own. He had learned about the free L.E.G.A.C.Y. neuropathy reversal workshops and made a decision to attend. He wasn't willing to give up. He had too much to live for. He dreamed of being the grandfather that could enjoy trips with his granddaughter and share smiles with her over their shared love of bluegrass music, history and the satisfaction that comes from building something

I

with your hands. But his failing health was putting all that in jeopardy.

Along with neuropathy, Elvin was suffering with back and neck pain from several bulging discs. He had lost noticeable function in his arms and legs. In addition, his balance was bad- one of the reasons he had to quit his career. He was taking numerous pharmaceuticals for his diabetes and high cholesterol. He was obese - at least 50 pounds overweight, adding extra wear and tear to his back and knees.

Elvin's story is heartbreaking, yet tragically common. His experience echoes the struggles of countless individuals grappling with neuropathy and its cascading effects on their lives. What began as a medical diagnosis had snowballed into a comprehensive assault on his physical, emotional, and social well-being. The dreams he held dear – of being an active, engaged grandfather – seemed now to be impossibly out of reach.

But Elvin's story is more than just a cautionary tale. It's a wake-up call, a stark reminder of the insidious nature of neuropathy and the urgent need for awareness, understanding, and effective interventions. His decision to attend the L.E.G.A.C.Y. workshop, despite the bleak prognosis he'd received, speaks to the resilience of the human spirit and the power of hope in the face of adversity.

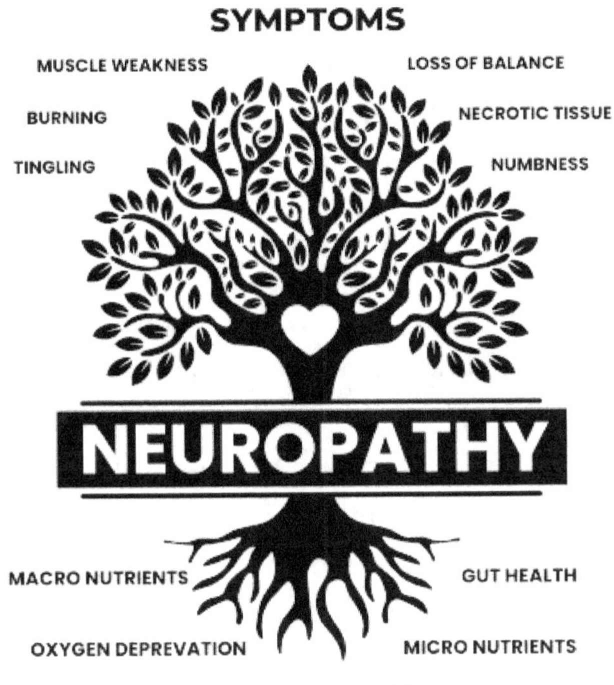

A quiet but urgent challenge is emerging in our communities. It starts with subtle signals—a slight numbness, a gentle tingle, or an occasional warm sensation. These signs might be easy to dismiss as fleeting or harmless, but they are early indicators of something more: neuropathy. This condition is becoming increasingly common in our modern world. By recognizing these signals and taking timely action, we have the power to address the root causes, regain control, and prevent neuropathy from progressing. Empowering our bodies through understanding and proactive care is the key to maintaining vitality and well-being.

Unveiling the Nerve Disruptor

Neuropathy, in its simplest terms, is a malfunction of your nerves. Think of your nerves as your body's electrical wiring, a vast network of communication lines carrying vital messages between your brain, spinal cord, and every other part of you. They control movement, sense touch and temperature, and even regulate all the stuff you don't have to think about- internal functions like digestion and heartbeat.

When neuropathy develops, it disrupts these signals. Now, Imagine frayed wires, faulty insulation, or short circuits in the system – messages get scrambled, garbled, or don't arrive at all. The result is a cascade of symptoms that can range from mildly irritating to completely life-altering.

The Many Faces of Neuropathy

Neuropathy doesn't show up the same way for

everybody.. Here are some common descriptions patients use to express their experiences:

- "Pins and needles" sensation in hands or feet
- Cold hands or feet
- Sharp, stabbing, or burning pain
- Extreme sensitivity to touch
- Weakness or clumsiness
- Muscle wasting or twitching
- Loss of balance and coordination

What Causes Neuropathy?

There are many different causes of neuropathy. Let's discuss some of the most common causes.

Diabetes

Diabetes is a chronic condition that affects how your body regulates blood sugar (glucose). When blood sugar levels become chronically elevated, it can damage various organs and tissues, including your nerves. This nerve damage is a major contributor to neuropathy.

Here's a breakdown of the main types of diabetes:

- **Type 1 Diabetes:** This autoimmune disease occurs when your body attacks the cells in your pancreas that produce insulin. Insulin is a hormone crucial for unlocking your cells and allowing them to absorb sugar from the bloodstream. Without enough insulin, sugar builds up in the blood, leading to the hallmark symptoms of diabetes.

- **Type 2 Diabetes:** This is the most common form of diabetes. In type 2 diabetes, your body either develops resistance to insulin's effects, or it doesn't produce enough insulin. This also leads to high blood sugar levels.
- **Gestational Diabetes:** This form of diabetes develops during pregnancy and usually resolves after childbirth. However, it can increase your risk of developing type 2 diabetes later in life.

If you're concerned about your risk of diabetes or neuropathy, a crucial first step is to check your blood sugar levels. Early detection and management of diabetes are essential to prevent complications like nerve damage. Here's how you can get started:

- **Talk to your doctor:** Discuss your risk factors and symptoms. They can advise you on the best approach for testing your blood sugar.
- **Consider home blood sugar monitoring:** With your doctor's guidance, you might use a

glucometer, a small device that allows you to easily check your blood sugar levels at home.

- **Start with small changes:** If your blood sugar levels are elevated, even minor adjustments to your diet and lifestyle can make a significant difference.

Remember, early detection and management are key. By taking charge of your blood sugar health, you can significantly reduce your risk of complications like neuropathy. The LEGACY program will be right here to support you every step of the way, providing resources and guidance to empower you on your journey towards optimal health.

Alcoholism

Chronic alcohol consumption is a significant risk factor for neuropathy. Alcohol damages your nerves in two main ways:

- **Direct Toxicity:** Alcohol itself is a neurotoxin, meaning it can directly damage the structure and function of your nerve cells. Imagine your nerves as delicate communication cables. Excessive alcohol acts like a poison, disrupting the signals traveling through these cables, leading to symptoms like numbness, tingling, and weakness.

- **Indirect Damage:** Alcohol disrupts the blood supply to your nerves. Think of your nerves like intricate electrical circuits. Healthy blood flow is crucial for delivering oxygen and essential nutrients to keep these circuits functioning properly. Alcohol damages the delicate lining of blood vessels, leading to restricted blood flow and depriving your nerves of the vital resources they need to thrive. This lack of oxygen and nutrients further contributes to nerve damage.

Excessive alcohol consumption also depletes your body's B vitamins, particularly B1 (thiamine) and B12. These B vitamins play a critical role in nerve health and function. Deficiencies in these vitamins can worsen neuropathy symptoms and lead to a condition called Wernicke-Korsakoff syndrome, known for causing memory problems, balance issues, and severe nerve damage.

If you're concerned about alcohol consumption and its impact on your nerves, the good news is that there's hope. Reducing or eliminating alcohol intake can significantly improve nerve health and potentially reverse some of the damage caused by alcohol.

Vitamin B12 deficiency

Vitamin B12 deficiency is a surprisingly common culprit behind neuropathy. This essential vitamin plays a critical role in maintaining the health and function of your nervous system. Here's how a B12 deficiency can contribute to nerve damage:

- **Protecting the Myelin Sheath:** Imagine your nerves as electrical wires. The myelin sheath acts like a fatty insulating layer surrounding these wires. It protects them and ensures smooth transmission of nerve signals. Vitamin B12 is crucial for the production and maintenance of this myelin sheath. When B12 levels are low, the myelin sheath becomes damaged, exposing the nerves and leaving them vulnerable to injury. This damage disrupts nerve signals, leading to symptoms like numbness, tingling, weakness, and pain.
- **B12 and Nerve Regeneration:** Beyond protection, vitamin B12 is also involved in nerve cell regeneration and repair. A deficiency can hinder your body's ability to repair damaged nerves, further worsening neuropathy symptoms.

So who's most at risk? Certain factors increase your risk of developing a B12 deficiency:

- **Diet:** Strict vegetarians and vegans are at higher risk, as B12 is naturally found in animal products like meat, poultry, fish, and eggs.
- **Age:** As we age, our ability to absorb B12 from food can decline.
- **Digestive Issues:** Conditions like Crohn's disease or pernicious anemia can interfere with B12 absorption.
- **Genetics:** Multiple genetic mutations can affect the body's ability to process and transport vitamin B12, including TCN1 and TCN2, MTHFR, FUT2, and Q5R just to name a few. An estimated 20% of individuals 60 years and older may have marginal vitamin B12 status.

If you suspect a B12 deficiency, a doctor can perform a simple blood test to confirm it. Treatment typically involves B12 supplements, which can be taken orally or through injections.

For those who can consume animal products, incorporating these B12-rich foods into your diet can be beneficial:

- Meat, poultry, and fish

- Eggs
- Dairy products
- Fortified foods like nutritional yeast

Remember: Always consult a doctor before starting any new supplements, especially if you have any underlying health conditions or are taking medications. The LEGACY program recognizes the importance of addressing B12 deficiency as part of our comprehensive approach to neuropathy management.

Autoimmune diseases

Autoimmune diseases are a group of conditions where your body's immune system, normally tasked with fighting off invaders like bacteria and viruses, mistakenly identifies healthy tissues as a threat. In some cases, this misplaced attack can target your nerves, leading to neuropathy. Here's a closer look at how autoimmune diseases can damage your nervous system:

- Certain autoimmune diseases, like Guillain-Barré syndrome and chronic inflammatory demyelinating polyneuropathy (CIDP), directly attack the nerves themselves. This attack can damage the myelin sheath, the protective layer surrounding nerves, or the nerves themselves. This disrupts nerve signaling, causing symptoms like weakness, numbness, tingling, and pain.

- Many autoimmune diseases involve chronic inflammation, a cellular firestorm that damages surrounding tissues. When nerves are caught in the crossfire of this inflammation, it can lead to nerve damage and neuropathy symptoms.

Examples of Autoimmune Diseases Affecting Nerves:

- **Guillain-Barré Syndrome (GBS):** A rapid onset of muscle weakness, often starting in the legs and spreading upwards, is a hallmark of GBS. This is caused by the immune system attacking the myelin sheath of peripheral nerves.
- **Chronic Inflammatory Demyelinating Polyneuropathy (CIDP):** Similar to GBS, but with a more gradual progression of weakness, numbness, and tingling.
- **Sjogren's Syndrome:** An autoimmune disease affecting the moisture-producing glands in your eyes and mouth. Some people with Sjogren's syndrome also experience neuropathy, likely due to damage to the small nerves in their hands and feet.

- **Lupus:** This systemic autoimmune disease can affect various organs, including the nervous system. Lupus-related neuropathy can cause a variety of symptoms, depending on which nerves are affected.
- Celiac disease: This disease is triggered by eating gluten, a protein found in wheat, rye, barley, and other grains. The body's immune system attacks the villi, which are tiny bumps that line the small intestine and help the body absorb nutrients.

If you have an autoimmune disease and experience any symptoms of neuropathy, it's crucial to seek medical attention promptly. Early diagnosis and treatment of the underlying autoimmune condition can help prevent further nerve damage and improve your quality of life.

Infections

Infections caused by viruses, bacteria, and even parasites can be surprising culprits behind neuropathy. These invaders can damage nerves directly or indirectly, leading to a range of symptoms like numbness, tingling, weakness, and pain. Here's a closer look at how infections can wreak havoc on your nervous system:

- Some infections, like Lyme disease caused by bacteria and shingles caused by the varicella-zoster virus (the same virus that causes chickenpox), directly target and damage nerve tissue. In the case of shingles, the virus can travel along nerve pathways, causing the characteristic painful rash and damaging the nerves themselves.

- Many infections trigger a robust immune response, leading to widespread inflammation. While this inflammation helps fight the infection, it can also damage surrounding tissues, including nerves. This collateral damage can disrupt nerve function and contribute to neuropathy symptoms.

Common Infectious Causes of Neuropathy:

- **Tick-borne illness:** Lyme disease and Bartonella, for example, can cause a variety of neurological symptoms, including neuropathy. The bacteria responsible for Lyme disease can directly infiltrate nerve tissue and cause inflammation, leading to nerve damage. Early and proper diagnosis and treatment of tick-borne infections are crucial to prevent long-term nerve damage.

- **Shingles**: This painful condition, characterized by a blistering rash, can also cause neuropathy. The varicella-zoster virus can travel along nerve pathways, damaging them and causing pain, numbness, and weakness in the affected area. Even after the rash clears, post-herpetic neuralgia, a form of neuropathy, can persist for months or even years.
- **HIV/AIDS**: The human immunodeficiency virus (HIV) can damage the nervous system in various ways, including causing neuropathy. HIV can directly infect nerve cells or indirectly damage them through the inflammatory response it triggers. Early diagnosis and treatment of HIV can help prevent or slow the progression of nerve damage.
- Other Infections: While less common, other infections like **cytomegalovirus (CMV)**, **Epstein-Barr virus (EBV)**, and some bacterial infections "like babesiosis" can also cause neuropathy.

If you suspect you might have an infection and experience symptoms of neuropathy, seeking prompt medical attention is crucial. Early diagnosis and treatment of the underlying infection can help prevent further nerve damage and improve your long-term prognosis.

Medications

Medications can play a vital role in treating various health conditions, but some can damage nerves directly or indirectly, leading to symptoms like numbness, tingling, weakness, and pain. Here's a breakdown of how certain medications can contribute to neuropathy:

- Chemotherapy drugs used to treat cancer are a prime example. These powerful medications work by targeting rapidly dividing cells, unfortunately, nerve cells can be susceptible. This damage to the nerve cells' DNA can lead to neuropathy.
- Certain antibiotics, particularly those from the class known as fluoroquinolones, can disrupt the production of myelin, the protective sheath surrounding nerves. This lack of myelin leaves the nerves vulnerable to damage and can contribute to neuropathy symptoms.
- Some studies show that certain statins used for lowering cholesterol actually increase the risk of neuropathy- simvastatin is commonly associated with muscle pain and weakness and atorvastatin is associated with a higher

incidence of polyneuropathy than other versions.

Other medications that can cause neuropathy:

- **Anticonvulsants:** Medications used to control seizures, like Gabapentin and Pregabalin, can sometimes cause numbness, tingling, or weakness as a side effect. This doesn't necessarily indicate neuropathy, but it's important to discuss these sensations with your doctor. Ironically, these drugs are very often prescribed to manage symptoms of neuropathy.
- **Pain medications:** Certain chronic pain medications, like Tricyclic antidepressants (TCAs) and some opioids, can cause numbness or tingling as a side effect.

Medications can be important, but it's crucial to weigh the benefits against potential side effects like neuropathy.

Physical injuries

Accidents happen, and sometimes those accidents can leave a lasting impact on your nervous system. Physical injuries, from car accidents and falls to sports injuries and repetitive stress, can be a significant cause of neuropathy. Here's how these injuries contribute to nerve damage:

- **Direct Nerve Compression or Laceration:** The most obvious scenario is a direct blow to a nerve. A car accident, fall, or even a deep cut can severely damage or sever a nerve, leading to immediate symptoms like numbness, weakness, and pain in the affected area.
- **Stretched or Pinched Nerves:** Even less dramatic injuries can cause neuropathy. Repetitive stress injuries, like carpal tunnel syndrome, occur when a nerve gets compressed or pinched by surrounding tissues. Over time, this compression can disrupt nerve function and lead to symptoms like tingling, numbness, and weakness.
- **Blood Vessel Damage and Starved Nerves:** Physical injuries can also damage blood vessels supplying nerves. These blood vessels deliver oxygen and essential nutrients to keep nerves healthy. If these blood vessels are damaged, the nerves become starved of these vital resources, leading to nerve dysfunction and potential neuropathy symptoms.

Examples of injuries leading to neuropathy:

- **Car accidents:** The force of a car accident can cause various injuries, including nerve damage. This can range from mild compression to complete nerve severance, depending on the severity of the accident.
- **Falls:** A fall, especially on an outstretched hand, can damage nerves in the wrist or arm. This can lead to carpal tunnel syndrome or other types of neuropathy.
- **Sports injuries:** Repetitive stress from certain sports can compress nerves, leading to neuropathy. For example, carpal tunnel syndrome is common in athletes who grip objects repeatedly, like cyclists and weightlifters.
- **Surgery:** While certain surgeries may be necessary, they can sometimes damage nerves during the procedure. This can lead to post-surgical neuropathy, causing numbness, pain, or weakness in the affected area.

If you experience an injury and develop symptoms like numbness, tingling, or weakness, seeking medical attention promptly is crucial. Early diagnosis and treatment of nerve damage can minimize long-term complications and improve your recovery.

Idiopathic neuropathy

Neuropathy can be like a detective story – sometimes the culprit is clear, but other times, the cause remains a puzzling mystery. Idiopathic neuropathy falls into this category. It refers to nerve damage where, despite extensive evaluation, no underlying reason can be identified. While idiopathic neuropathy is considered uncommon, being unable to determine the causes can be a significant source of frustration for those affected.

Here's a closer look at this enigmatic form of neuropathy:

- **Ruling Out the Usual Suspects:** Extensive testing for common causes like diabetes, vitamin deficiencies, autoimmune diseases, and infections is usually conducted. If all these come back negative, then idiopathic neuropathy becomes a possibility.
- **Far from being Unusual:** While uncommon, idiopathic neuropathy isn't exceptionally rare. It affects a significant portion -- 30-40% of neuropathy cases, making it an important piece of the neuropathy puzzle.

Even though the exact cause of idiopathic neuropathy remains elusive, there's still hope. Here's why:

- **Focus on What You Can Control:** While the cause might be a mystery, the focus can shift to managing symptoms and improving your quality of life. This can involve lifestyle modifications, targeted supplements, and pain management strategies.
- **Research on the Horizon:** Scientists continue to delve deeper into the potential causes of idiopathic neuropathy. Advances in research might someday shed light on the underlying mechanisms and lead to more targeted treatments.
- **We Often Win:** With the LEGACY model, its typical to see progress even if the specific cause is unknown. When we improve the health of the whole body, many things tend to improve. "A rising tide raises all ships" as the saying goes.

The LEGACY program acknowledges the challenges of navigating idiopathic neuropathy. We'll explore various strategies to support your nervous system health and empower you to become an active participant in your own wellness journey, even in the face of uncertainty.

If you have any of the risk factors for neuropathy, it's important to talk to your doctor about ways to reduce your risk of developing the condition. At Legacy Health, we have personalized, holistic treatments available to help you stop the progression and even reverse the process of neuropathy and improve your quality of life.

In simpler terms, a holistic approach means treating the whole you, not just the symptoms. It considers how different aspects of your life – your diet, stress levels, sleep patterns – can all work together to influence your neuropathy and your overall health. By addressing these various factors, we can create a personalized plan to improve your neuropathy and reclaim your quality of life.

The Price of Inaction: When Neuropathy Takes Its Toll

Too often, neuropathy's initial symptoms are downplayed or overlooked. This delay can have far-reaching consequences, both physically and emotionally. It's critical to understand the potential impact if neuropathy is left unaddressed, as this drives home the importance of early detection and action.

From Whisper to Whirlwind: Stories of Neuropathy Onset

- **Nancy's Fading Sensations:** Nancy's activities began to dwindle as numbness crept into her feet, devolving into a chronic "stuffiness" that dulled nearly half of her foot sensation. Walking became a challenge. Even simple pleasures like a stroll on the beach became distant memories. Her shoulder's range of motion decreased dramatically, further limiting her social life and even daily routines. As her neuropathy progressed, Nancy found herself increasingly disconnected from her community. She felt trapped in a body that seemed less and less like her own.

- **Diane's Frozen Feet:** The longer Diane dealt with neuropathy, the more she felt a persistent, icy sensation creeping in, making her feel as if her feet were perpetually frozen. Sleep was sparse as the discomfort kept her awake at night. Walking used to be automatic. Like many of us, she never even thought about it. Now, it's a daily struggle. As the neuropathy progressed, even short distances became daunting challenges, limiting Diane's independence and quality of life.

- **Mike's Vanishing Sensation:** Mike's world was rocked the longer he allowed his neuropathy to progress into his feet, particularly his right one. A gradual loss of sensation turned everyday activities into potential hazards, with driving becoming a nerve-wracking experience as he struggled to gauge his pressure on the pedals. He often wondered, "Should I even be doing this?!" Nighttime brought little respite, as shooting pains and leg cramps disrupted his sleep. Even his typical shoes became a source of discomfort. Wearing them for a single day would result in several days of regret. As the numbness progressed, Mike found himself questioning his ability to perform simple tasks safely. He found his independence slipping away with each passing day.

The Mounting Costs of Ignoring Neuropathy

Neuropathy's impact extends far beyond tingling and numbness. Ignoring its progression is like setting the stage for a cascade of consequences that can undermine your physical well-being, emotional resilience, and financial stability. It's a triple threat that demands our attention. Let's examine the far-reaching costs of inaction.

Physical Decline: The Body Struggles

- **From Discomfort to Debilitation:** While the initial tingling or prickling sensations may seem manageable, neuropathy often evolves. For many, these early symptoms can develop into persistent pain, muscle weakness, and a crippling loss of balance like it did for my dad. Imagine the difficulty of each step becoming a challenge or struggling with tasks that were once effortless, leading to a growing concern about maintaining independence.

- **Increased Risk of Injury:** Neuropathy weakens muscles and reduces coordination, increasing the likelihood of falls and fractures. Even minor accidents can have serious consequences, particularly when bones are fragile. These injuries can accelerate physical decline, creating a cycle of pain and immobility.

Emotional Toll: A Wounded Spirit

- **The Weight of Uncertainty:** Neuropathy brings with it many unknowns. Important questions linger: Will it get worse? How much of my abilities will I lose? How long will I be able to negotiate these stairs or manage my routine tasks? These uncertainties can lead to anxiety, as one worries about future limitations.

- **Coping with Pain and Loss:** Let's face it, chronic pain wears you down, both physically and mentally. Depression and feelings of isolation are common among those who feel paralyzed by their condition. Tasks once taken for granted become sources of frustration and despair, even eroding self-worth.

Financial Burden: The Cost of Care

- **The Spiraling Expenses:** Neuropathy treatment involves doctors' visits, diagnostic tests, medications, therapies, and potentially, assistive devices or wheelchairs. These costs add up quickly, especially considering that neuropathy is often a chronic condition requiring ongoing management.
- **Lost Income:** When neuropathy affects your ability to work, financial stress compounds. Disability benefits may provide some relief, but rarely replace your full income, creating a

significant gap that's hard to fill, especially when you're suffering.

- **Household Changes:** Severe neuropathy may necessitate home modifications like ramps, grab bars, stairlifts, or wider doorways. Some may even require assisted living. For those who are wheelchair-bound, it may require a move or adding an addition to their home. While essential for safety and independence, these adjustments represent another layer of financial burden.

Important Note: With my dad's condition, our family had to face every one of these aspects - physical, emotional, and financial. Understanding the potential consequences of ignoring neuropathy highlights the importance of early detection and proactive management.

Early Detection: Your Shield Against the Storm

The stories we've shared illustrate the potential consequences of neuropathy, but it's important to remember that there is always hope. Early diagnosis and proactive intervention are your greatest allies. By prioritizing early detection, you *significantly* increase the chances of slowing neuropathy's progression and preserving your quality of life. Here's how to tell when there's a problem::

- **Know the Signs:** Your body whispers long before it shouts. Take note of any unusual or persistent sensations, including:
    - Tingling or "pins and needles" in your hands, feet, or other areas
    - Numbness that diminishes your sense of touch
    - Burning, stabbing, or shooting pain
    - Weakness, especially in your legs or feet, leading to stumbling or tripping
    - Difficulty with balance or coordination
    - Unusual sensitivity to touch; hypersensitivity.
- **Seek a Qualified Professional:** If you suspect neuropathy, don't delay in finding a healthcare provider with specific experience in diagnosing and treating this complex condition. They are equipped to:
    - Conduct in-depth assessments, including functional nerve testing and other specialized diagnostics, to pinpoint the root cause of your neuropathy.
    - Develop a personalized treatment plan that addresses your specific needs and goals.

- Offer cutting-edge therapies and treatments that may not be widely available.

Important Addition: Our friendly team at Legacy Health is passionate about helping people find relief from neuropathy. We offer a compassionate, personalized approach, drawing from our extensive experience and advanced treatment options to help you reclaim your health and well-being.

- **Take Action:** Knowledge without action is meaningless- even harmful. If you suspect neuropathy, don't let fear or procrastination hold you back. Commit to the following:
  - Schedule an appointment with us as soon as possible. Don't hesitate to contact us at Legacy Health, 717-285-0001, or visit our website, getwellandstaywell.com. Even if you're not in our area, we have several colleagues around the country who may be able to offer support and help. Please remember that scheduling an appointment does not guarantee specific results.
  - Actively participate in your treatment plan. This may involve diet and lifestyle changes, nutrition, medication, physical medicine

approaches, and cutting-edge therapies tailored to your needs.

- ○ Embrace a proactive mindset. Neuropathy may be a part of your life, but it doesn't have to define it. Especially if dealt with early.

Remember, early detection is your most powerful weapon against neuropathy. By acting swiftly, you take control of your health and open the door to a brighter, symptom-free future.

The Painful Journey: When Neuropathy Progresses

Neuropathy isn't merely a physical ailment; it's a journey that takes a profound toll on body, mind, and spirit. While the path looks different for each individual, there are common threads of experience: escalating symptoms, a sense of diminishing control, and a profound emotional ripple effect. In this section, we'll explore the progression of neuropathy and the deeply personal stories of those who have faced it.

The Stages of Neuropathy: From Irritation to Devastation

While the pace of progression varies, neuropathy often

follows a pattern of worsening severity. Here's a simplified breakdown of potential stages:

- **Stage 1: Subtle Signs:** It often begins with nuisances that are easily dismissed – intermittent tingling, occasional numbness, or fleeting aches.
- **Stage 2: Intensifying Discomfort:** Symptoms transition from occasional to persistent. The tingling intensifies, numbness spreads, and pain becomes sharper – a constant companion interfering with daily life.
- **Stage 3: Functional Decline:** Weakness sets in, affecting balance, dexterity, and mobility. Simple tasks become frustrating ordeals, and the fear of falls is real and present danger.
- **Stage 4: Severe Debilitation:** In some cases, neuropathy progresses to excruciating pain, near-complete loss of sensation, and profound muscle weakness. Mobility may become severely compromised, and daily activities become insurmountable without assistance. There is usually some permanent nerve damage in this stage.

Important Note: Not everyone with neuropathy experiences all or even most of these stages. Early detection and treatment can significantly improve symptoms and quality of life for many individuals.

Voices from Those That Know

To truly grasp the impact of neuropathy, we must hear the voices of those who live with it every day. Here are a few examples:

- **Rick's Frozen Nights:** "My feet felt like blocks of ice all the time. I'd wake up five or six times a night. I wasjust trying to warm my feet. I tried everything to get them warm. Even an electric blanket didn't help – my nerves were so damaged, I couldn't even feel the heat. It was like living in constant winter- utterly exhausting"
- **Kathleen's Burning Isolation:** "For years, my feet were on fire. I couldn't wear socks or shoes. Even the lightest touch could be agonizing. I felt betrayed by my own body. I was unable to do simple things I once took for granted, simple things like walking. It was the worst I had felt in a decade."
- **Elsie's Electric Feet:** "For a couple of years, it felt like there were constant sparks in my feet. It was like walking on live wires all the time. I'd

been searching for some kind of relief for
years. It was easy to feel desperate and
hopeless at the same time- especially as my
foot pain persisted."

These stories offer a glimpse into the relentless physical pain, the erosion of independence, and the emotional anguish that neuropathy brings. Yet, even amidst this struggle, there is resilience. Understanding the process that develops this is the first step toward finding ways to win back our freedom.

The Emotional Toll: A Struggle Within

Neuropathy challenges you on two fronts – damaging your nerves while gradually limiting your freedom. The physical pain, loss of function, and increasing restrictions are clear hardships. Yet, beyond the physical, neuropathy also takes a profound emotional toll. Left unchecked, I've seen it diminish quality of life in subtle but serious ways. Let's examine these costs and explore how you can develop resiliency in your physical and mental health throughout this journey. Through modern science and the mind-body connections known about for centuries in ancient cultures, we know that emotions and stress hormones affect the organs and the brain chemistry.

- **Hopelessness and Despair:** Chronic pain, loss of independence, and the uncertainty of the future create a breeding ground for depression. Feelings of sadness, hopelessness, and loss of motivation are common among neuropathy patients. Despair and hopelessness affect the stomach, spleen, and pancreas. Stress in these areas can impact digestion and are associated with muscles that support the knees and back of the shoulders. The associated neurotransmitter, histamine, is related to inflammation, allergies and immune conditions.

- **Anxiety and Fear:** The constant worry about worsening symptoms, falls, or the need for more drastic interventions fuels anxiety. You might feel a loss of control and an impending doom about what lies ahead. These emotions can affect the kidney and bladder, bones, and spine and relate to Serotonin function. Stress in these areas can affect posture, back pain or disc problems because of the association with the hip flexors, back stabilizers and ankles.

- **Isolation and Loneliness:** Neuropathy symptoms can tempt you to withdraw from social activities you once loved. Pain, limited mobility, and embarrassment and confusion about your condition make it easier to stay home, leading to a sense of isolation that further compounds mental health struggles. The feeling of shame and others judging "what's wrong with you?" affect the brain and your vital energy sources. These emotions can affect the brain and central nervous system and relate to dopamine function. Shoulders and core stability are at risk of injury with the connection to the rotator cuff and abdominal muscles.

- **Anger, Resentment, and Frustration:** It's common to feel angry and frustrated with a condition that disrupts your life so profoundly. Resentment or bitterness are the most harmful. Emotions might be directed toward the medical system, your loved ones, yourself, or even God. These emotions can affect the liver and gallbladder and relate to the neurotransmitter Acetyl Choline which modulates muscle activation, memory and learning. Unresolved stress in these areas can inhibit shoulders and knees.

- There are many more correlations with stress and the physical effects on the body. If this mental-emotional aspect is ignored or undertreated, it's much more difficult to see lasting results.

The Physical Costs: A Body Out of Balance

- **Sleep Disruption:** The relentless pain of neuropathy can make sleep a nightmare. This lack of rest exacerbates pain sensitivity, weakens your immune system, and worsens mental health. A poor night's sleep has a 3 day blast radius. It takes around 72 hours for your immune system to recover. Additionally, the brain is unable to fully detoxify due to a faulty glymphatic system that operates normally when you sleep.
- **Decreased Activity:** Pain and fear of falling lead many neuropathy patients to become less active. This, unfortunately, accelerates muscle weakness and overall deconditioning, making symptoms worse over time. Inactivity diminishes vital input to the cerebellum, which is most known for its function with balance. We now know that the cerebellum also helps modulate and balance your emotional well-being.

- **Weight Fluctuations:** Changes in activity level, medication side effects, and emotional eating can lead to weight gain or loss, further impacting your overall health. Research indicates that for every pound of body weight, approximately 4 pounds of pressure is placed on weight-bearing joints like the back, hips and knees.

- **Weakened Immune System:** The combined stress of physical pain and emotional distress weakens your immune function, making you more susceptible to infections and slowing your body's healing ability.

Coping Strategies: Reclaiming Your Strength

While neuropathy presents challenges, it doesn't have to control your life. Here are strategies for safeguarding your physical and emotional well-being.

- **Seek Emotional Support:** Reach out to a doctor, therapist, or counselor certified in Neuro Emotional Technique. They can help reset the stress physiology driving many of these problems. They can also teach coping mechanisms for stress, anxiety, and depression. Support groups offer a sense of community and understanding.

- **Nurture Your Body:** Focus on healthy eating, gentle exercise (as tolerated), and prioritize sleep hygiene. Even small changes can make a difference in pain levels and energy.

- **Brain Training:** Techniques like practicing gratitude, deep breathing, or guided imagery calm the nervous system and offer moments of respite from pain and worry. These techniques, and more, can be tested by a qualified Applied Kinesiologist to help find the most personalized ones for your brain and nerve system.

- **Advocate for Yourself:** Be assertive with doctors, explore all treatment options, and don't settle for partial solutions. Your active participation is crucial. A great question to ask your providers is " If you were in my shoes, what would you do for yourself?'

- **Find Joy Where You Can:** Even amidst pain, seek out activities that still bring pleasure and meaning. Thoughts are powerful things. It takes the same amount of energy to think positive thoughts as it does negative ones. Creative hobbies, connecting with loved ones, or volunteering can be powerful antidotes to negativity.

Remember, you are not alone in this healing journey. By acknowledging the full impact of neuropathy and employing coping strategies, you can build resilience and maintain a sense of well-being even in the face of challenges.

When Neuropathy Takes a Devastating Turn

While the early signs of neuropathy may be easy to dismiss, delayed treatment or ineffective management can lead to a crisis point – a time when complications become severe, and everyday life is shattered. Understanding these potential consequences is a powerful motivator to seek effective solutions before it's too late.

When Neuropathy Becomes Critical: The Breaking Point

- **Falls and Injuries:** Weakened muscles, balance issues, and loss of sensation create a perfect storm for falls. These can lead to broken bones, head injuries, and a debilitating fear that restricts mobility and independence. This is the sad reality that me and my family lived through with my dad.
- **Non-Healing Wounds:** Neuropathy, especially in those with diabetes, impairs the body's

ability to heal wounds. Seemingly minor cuts on the feet can turn into dangerous ulcers and infections, with the risk of amputation looming in severe cases. I've seen more than I care to recount.

- **Complete Disability:** In some cases, neuropathy progresses to the point where walking becomes impossible, hand function is severely limited, and daily living tasks, like buttoning your shirt or pants become insurmountable. This level of disability is life-altering and requires significant support and care.

- **Unrelenting Pain:** For some, nerve pain takes on an excruciating quality that defies conventional medications. Just trying to function becomes all-consuming. It destroys sleep, eroding mental health, and tempts you to jettison the joy of life.

The Shortcomings of Conventional Neuropathy Treatments

It's a frustrating reality: countless neuropathy patients try traditional medical approaches only to find fleeting or disappointing results. While modern medicine offers many valuable tools, its approach to neuropathy often focuses on symptom suppression rather than addressing the root causes of the dysfunction. Let's dissect the key limitations of traditional treatments.

The Band-Aid Approach: Masking Pain, Not Solving Problems

- **Medication Overload:** The mainstay of conventional neuropathy treatment is prescription drugs, primarily those designed for other conditions. These may include:
  - **Antidepressants:** Used to alter pain perception in the brain, but they don't fix the underlying nerve damage. Also can be dangerous side effects- most school shootings were from people taking antidepressants.
  - **Anti-seizure medications:** They may offer temporary pain relief for some, but come with a host of side effects like dizziness, drowsiness, and cognitive impairment. Many of my patient's state "I feel like a zombie on that stuff."
  - **Opioids:** While sometimes prescribed for severe pain, they carry a high risk of addiction, worsen neuropathy over time, and don't address the root of the problem.

- **The Dangers of Dependence:** Long-term reliance on pain medication can lead to tolerance (requiring higher doses), addiction, and further health complications. Drugs are designed to mask your symptoms. It doesn't slow neuropathy's progression. It can't.

Missing the Big Picture: Incomplete Diagnosis

- **One-Size-Fits-All Diagnostics:** Conventional doctors often rely on limited testing methods like standard blood work and basic nerve conduction studies. These may detect some versions of neuropathy but often fail to reveal the specific type or the underlying factors driving it. Not to mention, they fail to give a useful treatment plan for improvement. They may help diagnose what's wrong, but rarely get to the PROCESS that is causing it to go wrong.
- **Treating Symptoms, Not Causes:** Without pinpointing the root cause or causes (diabetes, high histamine, nutrient deficiencies, toxins, heavy metals, infections etc.), treatment is guesswork. You may receive medication that masks pain temporarily, but the nerve damage itself continues unaltered.

Ignoring Mind-Body Connections: Medicine's Blindspot

- **Overlooking Stress:** Chronic physical and emotional stress wreaks havoc on your nervous system, exacerbating neuropathy symptoms. Yet, conventional medicine rarely addresses this crucial factor. And if they do, the treatment is commonly through more medications: anxiolytics or antidepressants.

- **Dismissive Attitudes:** Some doctors may dismiss your pain as age-related or minimize its impact. Many of my patient's have been told " you just have to learn to deal with it" This lack of empathy further compounds your frustration and sense of helplessness. You, the patient, should not be told "it's all in your head" or be blamed for their ignorance.

Important Note: This isn't to say that conventional medicine is useless. In some cases, medication may be necessary, especially for immediate pain relief. However, a comprehensive treatment plan must address the following:

- Identifying root causes through advanced diagnostics

- Treating the whole person, not just the symptoms
- Empowering patients with education and lifestyle change support

It's time to demand a better approach – one that seeks to heal, not just mask. In the following sections of this book, we'll explore real time-honored solutions that offer hope for long-lasting relief.

Case Studies

Here are just a few of the many case studies where conventional treatments failed when treating neuropathy:

- A 58-year-old man with diabetic peripheral neuropathy who did not respond to gabapentin, pregabalin, duloxetine, and tramadol[1].
- A 68-year-old man with diabetes and peripheral neuropathy who underwent a lumbar laminectomy and decompression for spinal stenosis. He did not experience any improvement in his lower extremity pain, numbness, and weakness after the surgery[2].
- A 67-year-old woman with chemotherapy-induced peripheral neuropathy who did not

benefit from amitriptyline, gabapentin, and pregabalin[3].

- A 72-year-old man with idiopathic peripheral neuropathy who failed to respond to amitriptyline, duloxetine, gabapentin, and oxycodone[4].

These case studies illustrate the frustrating reality that conventional treatments for neuropathy often provide inadequate or temporary relief. Diabetic neuropathy, post-surgical pain, chemotherapy-induced neuropathy, and even cases with unknown causes remain a challenge. This highlights the urgent need to change the conventional approach - It's time for approaches that address the root causes of nerve dysfunction and prioritize the individual patient's needs beyond symptom suppression.

Sources:

1. https://link.springer.com/article/10.1007/s12325-020-01462-3

2. https://diabetesjournals.org/clinical/article/19/3/122/2461/ Case-Study-A-68-Year-Old-Man-With-Diabetes-and

3. https://neurolrespract.biomedcentral.com/articles/10.1186/ s42466-020-00064-2

4. https://link.springer.com/content/pdf/10.1007/s12325-020-01462-3.pdf

The Hidden Dangers of Symptom Management: Why You Need More

While medications aimed at reducing pain may offer temporary relief, long-term reliance on them poses risks and misses the opportunity for true healing. It's essential to understand the potential downsides of this limited approach and why seeking solutions that address root causes is crucial for lasting improvement.

Risks of Symptomatic Treatment: The Price You Pay

- **Side Effects:** Every medication has a side-effect. Make sure you read the labels. Neuropathy medications carry a wide range of potential side effects, including:
  - Drowsiness or dizziness, which increases fall risk
  - Cognitive impairment or confusion
  - Nausea and digestive problems
  - Worsening of other health conditions
- **Dependence and Tolerance:** With long-term use of pain medications, your body may become tolerant, requiring higher doses for the same effect. This puts you in a higher risk

category for lIver and kidney damage. Dependence and even addiction can develop, creating a whole new set of problems. Not to mention that you are now an annuity for the drug companies!

- **Masking Progression:** While the pain is dulled, the underlying neuropathy can still worsen. This can lead to delayed diagnosis of serious complications or a false sense of security that the problem is under control.
- **Missed Opportunities:** Focusing solely on symptom suppression neglects other crucial aspects of your health that may be contributing to neuropathy, such as:
  - Nutritional deficiencies
  - Unmanaged blood sugar levels (if diabetic)
  - Toxic exposures
  - Stress and emotional burdens

Seeking Real Solutions: Pathways to Healing

- **Finding the Root Cause:** Thorough diagnostics are crucial – this may involve advanced blood tests, genetic screening, or specialized nerve function studies. Identifying the underlying cause empowers targeted treatments. Professional Applied Kinesiologists can be invaluable in this discovery process.

- **Addressing the Whole Person**: True healing considers all facets of your well-being:
  - **Nutrition**: Diet plays a major role in nerve health. Optimizing nutrient intake and addressing deficiencies is vital.
  - **Detoxification**: Identifying and reducing exposure to potential nerve toxins can be a game-changer for many patients. Again, manual muscle testing can be a useful tool, especially in discovering how the nerve system is reacting to a potentially toxic substance. Blood only measures what is transported, Urine and hair measure what is being excreted. In my opinion, the manual muscle test is unmatched in its sensitivity for determining toxic burdens on the nerves.
  - **Mind-Body Connection**: Stress management techniques, Applied Kinesiology, Neuro Emotional Technique, Quantum Neurology, EMDR, and other modalities help calm the nervous system, reset trauma responses and promote healing.

- **Innovative Therapies:** Explore options that go beyond conventional medicine:
  - Regenerative therapies that aim to stimulate nerve repair
  - Specialized physical therapy to improve balance and reduce fall risk
  - Photobiomodulation (light therapy), shown to decrease pain and promote nerve healing.

Disclaimer: Natural solutions aren't magic bullets. They often require commitment, patience, and an open mind. Always work with qualified healthcare professionals when exploring these options.

You have the power to advocate for a holistic treatment plan that addresses the root causes of your neuropathy and supports your long-term health. It's time to look beyond just managing symptoms and embark on a journey towards true healing.

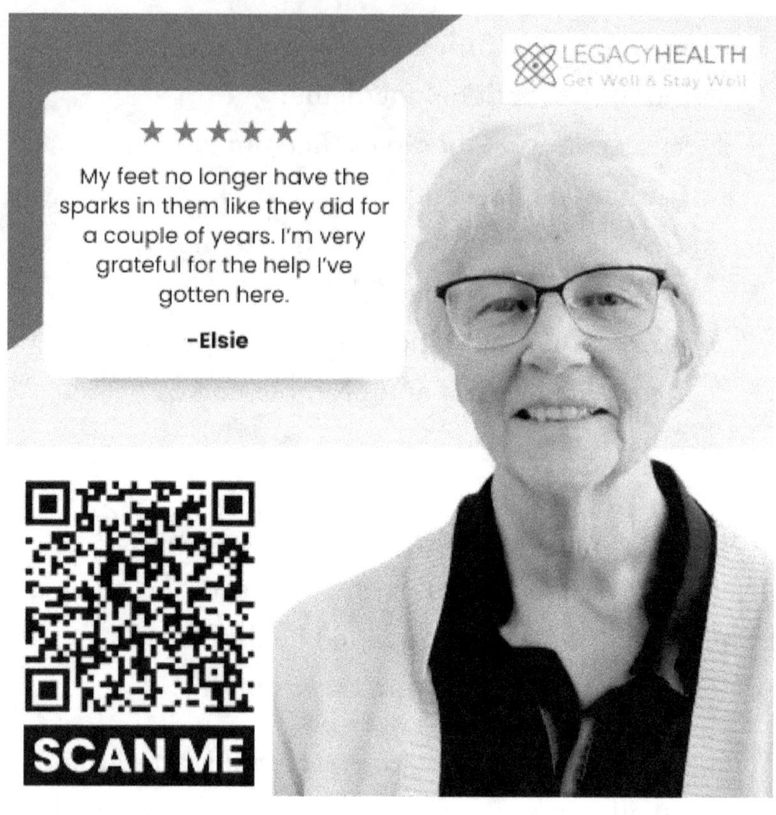

Unlock Your Path to Neuropathy Relief Now: Call 717-285-0001 to Speak With a Skilled Neuropathy Professional Today!

2

RECLAIMING YOUR LIFE: THE L.E.G.A.C.Y. NEUROPATHY SOLUTION

LEGACY

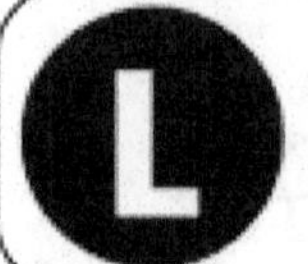 **L** isten Intently to Your Story 

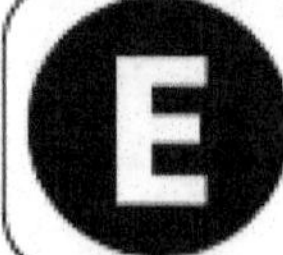 **E** xpert Efficient Exam 

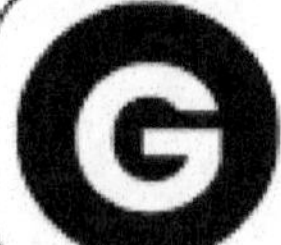 **G** entle Genius Protocols 

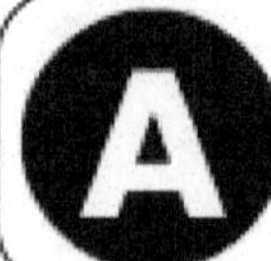 **A** ctivate Healing Response 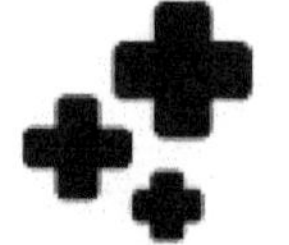

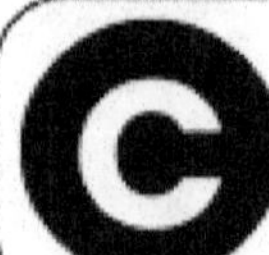 **C** reate Mind-Body Connections 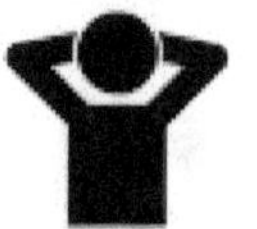

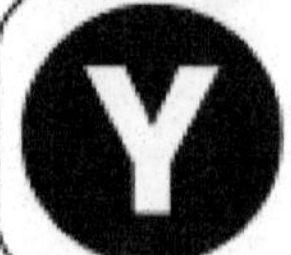 **Y** our Legacy Now, You Only Live Once! 

If you're battling neuropathy, you may feel like you've tried everything. Pills that numb the pain but don't fix the problem. Doctors who offer vague explanations and limited solutions. The frustration and despair can be overwhelming. But it's time for a new approach, a brighter path forward – it's time for L.E.G.A.C.Y.

Introducing the L.E.G.A.C.Y. Neuropathy Program

The L.E.G.A.C.Y. Neuropathy Program is a revolutionary system designed to go beyond mere symptom management and address the root causes of your nerve distress. It's a comprehensive approach rooted in the understanding that true healing requires addressing all aspects of your health. Let's break down what L.E.G.A.C.Y. stands for:

- L - Listen Intently to Your Story: Your journey is unique. We start by truly listening to your experiences, concerns, and goals. This deep understanding guides your personalized treatment plan.
- E - Expert Efficient Exams: We utilize cutting-edge diagnostic tools and thorough evaluations to pinpoint the underlying factors contributing to your neuropathy. When necessary, this goes far beyond the standard medical tests.

- **G** - Gentle Genius Protocols: We harness the power of advanced therapies, gentle techniques, and proven protocols to target nerve dysfunction at its source, promoting regeneration and restoring function.
- **A** - Activate Healing Response: Your body has an innate ability to heal. Our treatments are designed to stimulate your natural healing mechanisms, optimizing nerve health and overall well-being.
- **C** - Create Mind-Body Connections: Your mind and body are deeply connected. We'll teach you tools and techniques to reduce stress, calm your nervous system, and promote an environment conducive to healing.
- **Y** - Your Legacy Now, You Only Live Once! Neuropathy doesn't have to define your life. We're committed to helping you reclaim your health, your vitality, and write a new chapter filled with joy and possibility.

The L.E.G.A.C.Y. program is not a quick fix or a one-size-fits-all solution. It's a journey of transformation, tailored to your individual needs and guided by a dedicated team committed to helping you achieve your health goals.

Beyond Pills and Procedures: The Power of a Holistic Approach

Traditional medicine often falls short in treating neuropathy because it treats the symptom (pain) rather than the person as a whole. A holistic approach recognizes that your body is more than the sum of its parts and systems. It is an interconnected matrix, and that your neuropathy is likely the result of multiple factors, not just a single malfunction. This comprehensive perspective is your key to lasting relief and improved overall well-being.

Benefits of a Holistic Approach

- **Root-Cause Resolution:** Instead of merely masking pain, a holistic approach aims to identify and address the underlying drivers of your neuropathy, such as:
    - Nutritional deficiencies
    - Inflammation
    - Allergies and Sensitivities
    - Toxic exposures
    - Genetic weaknesses
    - Electrical Pollution
    - Chronic Infections
    - Unmanaged blood sugar (in diabetics and pre-diabetics)

- ○ Hormonal imbalances
- ○ Structural problems
- ○ Emotional stress
- **Tailored Treatment:** No two cases of neuropathy are alike. A holistic approach means personalized treatment plans that are based on your unique needs and goals,
- **Whole-Person Healing:** True healing extends beyond physical symptoms. Holistic care addresses factors like stress management, emotional well-being, and lifestyle modifications, leading to improved quality of life in all aspects.
- **Long-Term Results:** By tackling the root causes of neuropathy and optimizing your overall health, a holistic approach can lead to lasting improvements and reduce the risk of complications down the road.

Promises of the L.E.G.A.C.Y. Neuropathy Program

The LEGACY system embodies the principles of holistic care. Here's what you can expect:

- **Finding the "Why":** We go beyond generic diagnoses, using advanced testing to uncover the specific factors contributing to your neuropathy- Structural, Metabolic and

Emotional. This knowledge empowers us to create a targeted treatment plan.

- **Treating the Whole You:** Our program incorporates therapies that directly address nerve dysfunction alongside strategies to enhance overall well-being. This could include nutritional guidance, detoxification support, stress reduction techniques, and specialized therapies.

- **Empowering You:** We don't just treat you; we educate you. Understanding your condition empowers you to make positive lifestyle changes that support long-term healing.

- **A Partnership for Success:** Your active participation in your treatment is key. We'll work as a team, providing guidance, support, and accountability as you journey towards lasting relief.

The LEGACY program is a commitment to finding solutions that work for you, not just covering up the problem. It's about helping you reclaim your health, your freedom, and your joy in life.

Transformative Healing: Reversing Neuropathy, Reclaiming Your Life

Neuropathy can feel like an impossible challenge, slowly eroding your quality of life. Yet, the LEGACY program offers a different path. Through comprehensive treatment targeting the root causes of your condition, true healing is possible. Don't just take our word for it – let's hear the voices of transformation.

The Power of Comprehensive Treatment

While each patient's journey is unique, the LEGACY system consistently delivers meaningful results by addressing the multifaceted nature of neuropathy. Here's how our comprehensive approach often leads to significant improvements:

- **Reduced Pain and Discomfort:** Advanced therapies, combined with optimizing nerve health from our Applied kinesiology approach, can dramatically decrease the burning, tingling, and numbness that plague patient's suffering with neuropathy.
- **Improved Balance and Mobility:** By addressing the brain, muscle weakness, sensory issues, and underlying structural problems, patients often regain significant

stability, reducing the risk of falls and increasing confidence in their movements.

- **Enhanced Sleep and Energy**: When pain is reduced and the nervous system is calmed, restful sleep returns. This translates to better energy levels and overall well-being throughout the day.
- **Beyond Physical Healing**: Many patients experience improved mood, reduced stress levels, and a renewed sense of optimism as their healing progresses. I commonly hear " I just feel better all over! "

Testimonials: Transformation in Their Own Words

- **Leroy's Renewed Mobility**: "My legs and hands were burning and tingling, making it hard to walk or even keep my balance. But now, thanks to the L.E.G.A.C.Y. program, it's like my legs are waking up! The pain is much less, and I'm finally regaining my mobility."
- **Sandy's Steps to Freedom**: "I've seen a lot of progress with my neuropathy. When I first came in, I was in pretty bad shape and couldn't walk. I experienced a lot of pain in my legs. But now, my right leg is pain-free, and my left leg is feeling better. The

treatment is helping, and it's worth every penny."

- **Elsie's Sparkling Relief:** "My feet no longer have the sparks in them like they did for a couple of years. It was well worth the hour and a quarter drive I made for my appointments. I'm very grateful for the help that I've gotten here."

These testimonials highlight the potential of the LEGACY program. Individual results may vary, but they represent the hope and transformation that are possible with the right treatment approach.

Are you ready to experience your own transformation?

Embracing Your Healing Journey: Take the First Step

You've learned about the devastating impact of neuropathy, the limitations of traditional treatments, and the promise of the LEGACY program. Now, it's time to move from knowledge to action. If you're ready to break free from the grip of neuropathy and start building a healthier, symptom-free future, the path is open to you.

Your Transformation Starts Here

We're here to guide you every step of the way. Here's how to begin:

- **Schedule Your Consultation:** Take charge of your health! Call Legacy Health at 717-285-0001 or visit getwellandstaywell.com/contact to schedule your appointment. This is your chance to have your questions answered, explore your options, and start crafting your personalized treatment plan. Please note that while we strive to provide the best possible care for our patients, a consultation does not guarantee specific results. We'll work with you to determine if the LEGACY program is a good match for your individual needs.

- **Attend Our Informative Workshop:** Want to learn more before your consultation? Reserve your seat at our next in-person workshop by texting "PAIN FREE" to 717-987-7820. Discover the root causes of neuropathy, the power of the LEGACY system, and hear inspiring success stories from other patients. We often do a live demonstration of some of the therapies so you can experience some transformation in real time. This workshop is for educational purposes only and does not constitute medical advice. Individual results with the LEGACY program may vary.

Why Choose Legacy Health?

- **Leading-Edge Therapies:** We're committed to providing our patients with access to the most advanced neuropathy treatments available, including therapies and techniques that may not be offered elsewhere.
- **Personalized Care:** Your journey is unique, and your treatment plan will be too. We take the time to understand your specific needs and goals.
- **Compassionate Team:** We understand the struggles of neuropathy and are genuinely invested in your success. You'll find support and encouragement every step of the way.

Don't give neuropathy control your life any longer. The power to heal lies within you – let us help you unleash it. Contact us today to start your transformation!

Beyond Symptom Management: Targeting the Root of Your Neuropathy

Traditional medicine often focuses on numbing the pain of neuropathy or masking its symptoms. While this might offer temporary relief, it doesn't address the underlying factors driving the nerve damage. To achieve lasting improvement, we must dig deeper and treat the causes, not just the consequences.

Addressing Root Causes: The Key to Lasting Change

Here's where the LEGACY approach diverges from conventional treatment:

- **Thorough Diagnostics:** We utilize advanced testing to pinpoint the specific drivers of your neuropathy. This might include:
    - Bloodwork to assess nutritional status, inflammation markers, allergies , hidden infections and blood sugar levels
    - Genetic testing to identify predisposition to certain types of neuropathy
    - Hair or Urine testing to assess toxic body burdens
    - Micro-Circulation Screening to check your blood flow

- ○ Digital Balance Tests to quantify your fall risk
  - ○ Specialized nerve function studies
- **Individualized Treatment:** Based on your diagnostic findings, we create a plan that may include:
  - ○ Nutritional support to correct deficiencies that impair nerve health
  - ○ Detoxification protocols to reduce exposure to nerve-damaging toxins
  - ○ Therapies for structural imbalances that can alter nerve transmission
  - ○ Stress management techniques to reset an overtaxed nervous system
  - ○ Regenerative therapies to promote nerve repair

Comparative Examples: Symptom Relief vs. Root-Cause Resolution

Let's illustrate the difference with a few hypothetical examples.

Scenario 1: Diabetic Neuropathy

- **Symptom Management:** Prescribing pain medication to mask foot pain.

- **Root-Cause Approach:** Blood sugar optimization through diet and lifestyle changes, plus therapies to improve circulation and nerve health.

Scenario 2: Vitamin Deficiency

- **Symptom Management:** Pain medication or nerve-calming drugs.
- **Root-Cause Approach:** Identifying and correcting the specific vitamin deficiency (e.g., B12), combined with therapies to support nerve repair.

Scenario 3: Post-Surgical Neuropathy

- **Symptom Management:** Relying on pain medication for ongoing discomfort.
- **Root-Cause Approach:** Specialized therapies to reduce inflammation, release scar tissue, and restore proper nerve function.

Important Note: Even if traditional medication is necessary in the short term, the LEGACY system always prioritizes identifying and addressing the root causes to break the cycle of pain and dysfunction.

True healing means looking beyond the obvious and treating the whole person.

The Power of Root-Cause Healing: Why It's Your Best Option

While medications may have their place in managing neuropathy symptoms, they often provide a flimsy temporary band-aid rather than a long-term solution. Root-cause healing, on the other hand, addresses the underlying dysfunction driving your symptoms. Let's examine why this approach is key to your lasting well-being.

Advantages Over Symptomatic Care

- **Sustainable Results:** Targeting the root causes of neuropathy offers the potential to slow or reverse its progression, reduce your reliance on medication, and achieve lasting relief.
- **Reduced Side Effects:** neuropathy drugs come with a risk of side effects and complications. Finding and treating the root cause minimizes the need for long-term medication use. It's not uncommon for my patients to reduce or eliminate their use of medications.
- **Proactive Prevention:** By addressing factors like nutritional imbalances or inflammation,

root-cause healing lessens the risk of neuropathy complications down the road.

- **Improved Overall Health:** True healing is never just about one symptom. Root-cause treatment often leads to better sleep, improved energy, and a greater sense of well-being throughout your life.

How to Embrace Root-Cause Healing

- **Find a Practitioner Who Understands Neuropathy:** When seeking care for neuropathy, it's essential to find a healthcare provider with experience in this complex condition and a focus on functional medicine, which seeks to address the root causes of illness. Practitioners trained in Applied Kinesiology, for example, are often skilled in looking beyond surface symptoms to identify the underlying factors contributing to your neuropathy.

- **Be Patient and Committed:** Root-cause healing doesn't offer overnight miracles. It requires a commitment to the treatment process and necessary lifestyle changes. But most patients are surprised by how quickly their body can actually heal.

- **Focus on Progress, Not Perfection:** Even small improvements are significant steps towards lasting relief. Celebrate your wins (without inflammatory foods) and stay motivated on your journey.
- **Become an Active Participant:** The most successful patients ask questions, educate themselves about their condition, and are proactive in supporting their healing.

Remember: Masking symptoms only prolongs the problem. Root-cause healing offers the chance of a better future – a life where neuropathy doesn't hold you back.

The Journey to Get Well: Your Path to Reclaiming Your Life

The LEGACY program is more than just a collection of treatments – it's a journey of healing and empowerment. While everyone's experience is unique, there are common milestones and key phases along the way. Let's explore what you might expect, reinforced by the voices of those who have walked this path before you.

The Path of the LEGACY Neuropathy Program

- **Phase 1: Discovery and Understanding:** Your journey begins with a comprehensive consultation and thorough diagnostic workup. We listen to your story, identify potential root causes, and create a personalized treatment plan.

- **Phase 2: Targeting the Source:** This phase involves targeted therapies to address your specific needs. Applied Kinesiology helps direct your personalized care. This might include nutritional support, individualized food plan, regenerative or detox treatments, stress reduction techniques, specialized physical therapy, or a combination of approaches.

- **Phase 3: Experiencing Results:** As your body responds to treatment, you'll likely notice increased muscle function and mobility. Some are gradual improvements and some are dramatic and immediate. Pain may lessen, energy levels may rise, and you may start to regain lost function. This progress fuels your motivation.

- **Phase 4: Empowerment and Maintenance:** We teach you how to support your ongoing healing through lifestyle changes, at-home exercises, and self-care strategies. You gain the tools to manage your condition long-term.

Patient Journey Stories: Transformations in Action

- **Elvin's Renewed Hope**: "My medical doctors told me I'd be in a wheelchair in 10 years, and they couldn't do anything for me but pain medicine. And now I have some hope. I can play with my grandkids again. I'm impressed with how this program is working."
- **Karen's Simple Joys**: "My feet are not burning. I can put shoes on. I can wear socks. Things I could never do before. It is the best I have felt in 10 years."
- **Rich's Whole-Body Healing**: "Dr. Tomasetti is always my first choice of doctor to call about many different situations, not simply spinal adjustment. His knowledge of the intricate workings of the human body and mind allows him to get to the root of a problem, not simply give a temporary relief of pain. Ten stars if I could!"

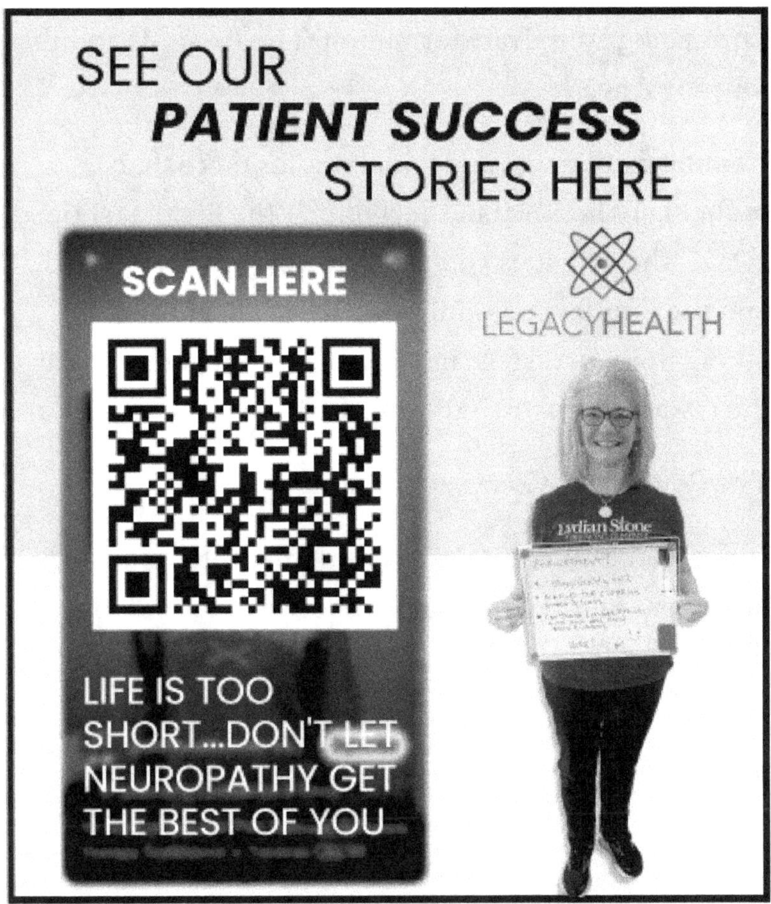

Important Note: Individual results vary, and healing is not always linear. There may be ups and downs, but our team is here to support you every step of the way.

The LEGACY program is a partnership. We provide the guidance; you bring the determination – together, we create lasting change.

Embracing Your Transformation: The Rewards and the Journey Ahead

Healing from neuropathy is about far more than reducing pain. It's about reclaiming the life that slipped away – the activities you miss, the joy you abandoned, and the limitless possibilities that lie ahead. While taking those first steps might feel daunting, know that the rewards are worth the effort.

The Rewards of Complete Healing

Close your eyes and take a few moments to Imagine a life where neuropathy is no longer your central focus. Seriously, I'll wait here for a bit. Here's what most of my patients experience:

- **Reduced Pain and Improved Function:** Less pain, tingling, and numbness mean better mobility, balance, and an ability to reclaim daily tasks and hobbies.
- **Restful Sleep and Renewed Energy:** When pain doesn't dominate your nights, you wake refreshed. This translates to better energy levels and mental clarity throughout the day. If you're like me, you're not as edgy with your loved ones when you're well rested.
- **Emotional Well-being:** Chronic pain takes a toll on your mental health. As healing

progresses, many find their mood lifting, anxiety or depression decreasing, and a renewed sense of optimism.

- **Rediscovering Your Potential**: Neuropathy can limit you in unexpected ways. With improved health, you may have the energy and confidence to pursue activities, goals, or relationships that previously fell out of reach.

Preparing for the Journey

Embarking on the path to healing takes courage and commitment. Here's how to set yourself up for success:

- **Mindset Matters**: Believe in your body's ability to heal. Your body knows just what to do, it simply needs no interference to the healing process. Embrace a mindset of grace, patience, persistence, curiosity and self-compassion.
- **Support System**: According to a report by the Health Resources and Services Administration, loneliness and social isolation can be as damaging to health as smoking 15 cigarettes a day. This highlights the severe impact of relationships on physical health. Surround yourself with people who believe in you. Ask for help when needed, and share your

successes with those who celebrate your progress.

- **Open Communication:** Be an active participant in your treatment. Ask questions, share your concerns, and keep your healthcare team updated on any changes you experience.
- **Celebrate Milestones:** Keep a gratitude journal. This can be helpful when things get bumpy- a good reminder of what's truly important. Healing isn't always a straight line. Acknowledge even small improvements and use them as fuel to keep moving forward.

The journey to wellness may have its challenges, but the rewards are immeasurable. By choosing to address the root causes of your neuropathy, you choose to invest in a future filled with vitality, freedom, and the boundless possibilities that come with true health.

Tired of endless medications that just mask your neuropathy pain? Ready to find lasting relief and reclaim your life? Take the first step towards healing! Call Legacy Health at 717-285-0001 or visit getwellandstaywell.com/contact to schedule your appointment. While we strive to provide effective treatment options, individual results may vary, and we cannot guarantee specific outcomes.

Want to learn more first? Text "PAIN FREE" to 717-987-7820 to reserve your seat at our next workshop and discover the root causes of neuropathy and how to break free. This workshop is intended for educational purposes only and does not constitute medical advice. It is not a guarantee of specific results.

ACTION STEP: Start a daily journal of your symptoms. This will allow you to more accurately sense your level of improvement when starting a neuropathy treatment regimen.

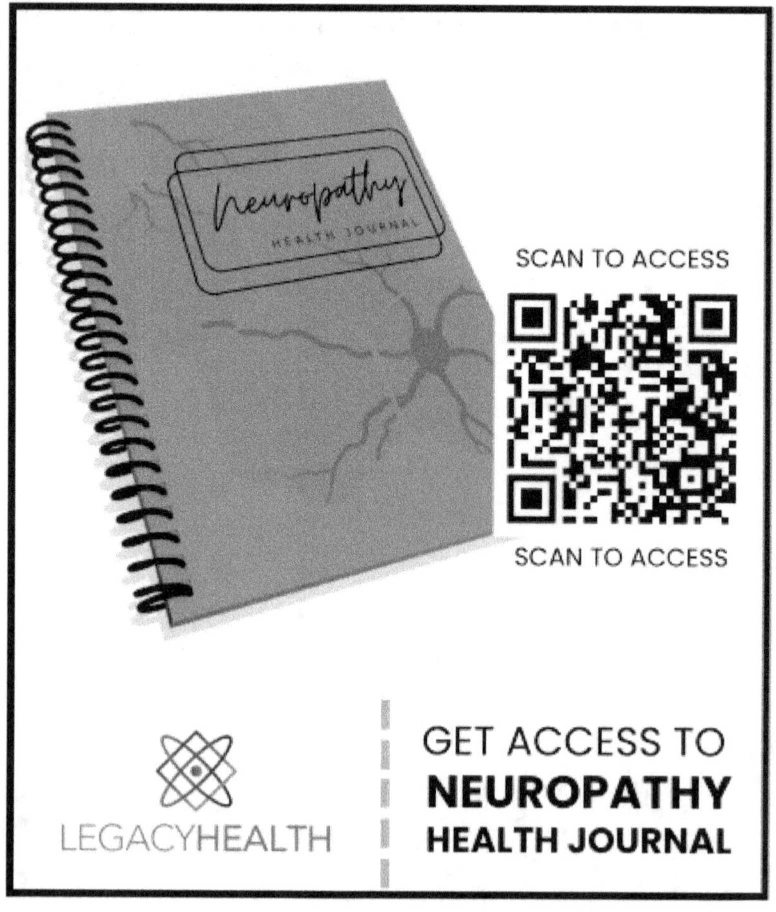

Unlock Your Path to Neuropathy Relief Now: Call 717-285-0001 to Speak With a Skilled Neuropathy Professional Today!

3

———

NEUROPATHY TRUTHS: EXPOSING THE MYTHS, EMPOWERING YOUR HEALING

Sadly, the world of neuropathy treatment is soaked with half-truths, unsubstantiated claims, and outright falsehoods. These myths create false hope, lead to wasted resources, and can even delay you from finding solutions that truly work. Let's debunk five of the most common myths and arm you with the knowledge you need to make informed decisions.

Myth #1: "Neuropathy only affects people with diabetes."

Why It's Dangerous

- **Missed Diagnoses:** This misconception leads those with neuropathy, but without diabetes, to dismiss their symptoms. This delays the diagnosis of other serious conditions that need to be improved (e.g., autoimmune disease or vitamin deficiencies).

- **Narrow Treatment Focus:** If doctors believe neuropathy is always diabetes-related, they may overlook potential root causes and treatments that would be more effective for the individual patient.
- **Heightened Anxiety for Diabetics:** While diabetic neuropathy is a serious concern, this myth creates unnecessary fear in those newly diagnosed with diabetes – they may think nerve damage is inevitable, when it's often preventable. In fact, with the right treatment, most type 2 diabetes is reversible.

Reality Check

- **Diverse Causes:** Let's emphasize the range of potential neuropathy triggers:
    - **Nutrient Deficiencies:** Especially Essential Fatty Acids, VitaminB12, B1, B6 and Vitamin D, which are vital for nerve health. Testing for these should be a standard part of neuropathy workups.
    - **Autoimmune Diseases:** Rheumatoid arthritis, lupus, Raynaud's, Scleroderma

and others can attack nerves. Controlling inflammation and addressing the underlying condition is crucial.

- **Injuries/Surgeries:** Even old injuries can cause nerve dysfunction, compression or damage. Specialized therapies and trauma repatterning can release these restrictions and promote healing.
- **Toxins:** Heavy metals, chemicals in cosmetics and weed killers, molds and even excessive alcohol use – identifying and removing these exposures is vital for some patients.
- **Medication Side Effects:** Certain chemotherapy drugs, antibiotics, statins and others. Sometimes, medication adjustments can make a major difference.
- **Unexplained Cases:** Sadly, there are times when even with thorough testing, a definitive cause or causes isn't found. This doesn't mean nothing can be done - targeting symptom relief and nerve support remain key.

The Takeaway: While diabetes IS a major neuropathy risk factor, it's never the assumed culprit. There are over a hundred known causes of neuropathy in the literature. A thorough investigation to uncover ALL potential root causes is needed for both diabetics AND non-diabetics with neuropathy.

Myth #2: "I've heard, 'Nerves don't regenerate.'"

Why It's Outdated:

This myth stems from a time when our understanding of nerve regeneration was limited. Here's why it's no longer accurate:

- **Peripheral vs. Central Nervous System:** It's true that nerve cells (neurons) in the central nervous system (brain and spinal cord) have very limited regenerative abilities, but they can create workarounds. This ability, known as neuroplasticity, allows your brain to form new connections and pathways, much like building new roads or enhancing existing ones for smoother travel. It's this adaptability that enables learning, recovery, and personal growth throughout your life. Incorporating the principles of applied kinesiology, we can further harness neuroplasticity by finding and using specific physical movements and exercises to stimulate the brain's natural reorganization. This approach taps into the body-brain connection, encouraging the development of healthier habits, improving physical well-being, and even aiding in the recovery from head injuries or strokes. Essentially, applied kinesiology offers a roadmap for guiding the brain's adaptability to enhance our overall health and function. However, the peripheral nervous system is different!

- **The Role of Schwann Cells:** The peripheral nerves are wrapped in a protective sheath made up of cells called Schwann cells. These cells play a crucial role in regeneration by guiding and supporting the new growth of nerve fibers.
- **Factors Affecting Regeneration:** While regeneration depends on the severity of damage, factors like the person's age, overall health, and targeted therapies can greatly impact the process.

Reality Check: The Potential for Nerve Healing

- Research Advances: Numerous studies demonstrate that with the right support, peripheral nerves can regenerate and regain function. This opens up new avenues for treating neuropathy.

- Regenerative Therapies: Emerging therapies focus on stimulating nerve repair, some of which include:
    - Specialized forms of light therapy
    - Digital Electrictro Therapeutic nerve stimulation
    - Nutritional support (B vitamins, omega-3 fatty acids, etc.)
    - Targeted anti-inflammatory and circulatory supplementation
- Optimizing Your Healing Environment: Reducing inflammation, managing blood sugar, and adopting stress-reduction techniques can all create a more conducive environment for nerve regeneration.

The Takeaway: While nerve regeneration may not always be a quick or complete process, it's far from impossible. In fact we see it happen all the time. Dismissing this potential leaves patients feeling hopeless when there may be options to restore function and improve their quality of life.

Myth #3: "I only have sporadic numbness and tingling, so it's no big deal."

Why It's Dangerous

- **Progressive Nature:** Neuropathy often worsens slowly over time. The early tingling may spread or intensify, and the numbness can progress to a loss of sensation. Pain might develop, ranging from mild discomfort to unbearable burning or sharp sensations.

- **Increased Risk of Injury:** Decreased sensation and numbness in your feet and hands makes you vulnerable to falls, burns, and unnoticed cuts that can lead to serious infections. Muscle weakness can further increase fall risk.

- **Loss of Independence:** As balance worsens and pain increases, simple tasks like walking or dressing can become a painful challenge. This may erode independence and quality of life. Some patients lose their ability to drive or even walk unassisted.

- **Delayed Treatment is Costly:** Early intervention can significantly slow progression and reduce the risk of long-term complications. Ignoring it means missed opportunities for potential improvement, and may lead to more expensive, invasive or permanent treatments down the road.

Reality Check: Catching the Fire Early

- **Listen to Your Body:** Numbness and tingling are NOT normal. They are your body's alarm system signaling nerve damage.
- **Gradual Doesn't Mean Trivial:** Even if your symptoms feel mild right now, don't assume they always will be. Early diagnosis allows for proactive steps to protect yourself.
- **The Ripple Effect:** Neuropathy can impact every aspect of your life: from mobility, to sleep, to emotional well-being. Treating it early minimizes this disruption.

The Takeaway: Dismissing those early signs is like ignoring a smoldering fire – before you know it, it can engulf your life and those you are responsible to support. Seeking help early on is the best way to prevent neuropathy from digressing to permanant nerve damage and forcing you and your loved ones to make difficult decisions about your health and well-being. Don't wait to get checked!

Myth #4: "Neuropathy is a natural result of aging."

Why It's Harmful

- **Missed Opportunities:** If this were true, then everyone would develop neuropathy symptoms within a certain age range- this doesn't happen. This misconception leads people to accept pain and dysfunction as normal, causing them to miss out on treatments that could substantially improve their quality of life.
- **Ageism and Self-Neglect:** It reinforces a negative mindset about aging, making people less likely to advocate for their health and explore solutions for their neuropathy.
- **Masking Deeper Issues:** Dismissing neuropathy as "age-related" delays diagnosis of underlying conditions (diabetes, vitamin deficiencies, etc.) that need management to prevent further complications.

Reality Check: Aging Doesn't Guarantee Neuropathy

- **Nerve Changes vs. Dysfunction:** While some age-related changes in the nerves are common, they don't automatically lead to debilitating neuropathy.
- **Lifestyle Factors Matter:** Many older adults maintain healthy nerve function due to:

- ○ Good nutrition
- ○ Managed blood sugar
- ○ Staying active
- ○ Addressing underlying health conditions proactively
- **Preventive Potential:** Even for those with neuropathy risk factors due to age, it's never too late to take action. Optimizing diet, blood sugar control, and adopting nerve-supportive therapies can make a significant difference. I've even had patients in their late 80's and 90's make major improvements.

The Takeaway: Neuropathy is NOT a mandatory part of the aging process. By proactively managing your health and addressing any developing nerve symptoms, you can protect yourself and preserve your quality of life as you age.

Myth #5: "I have to accept my neuropathy and learn to live with it."

Why It's Disempowering

- **Reinforces Despair:** This myth is typically perpetuated by well-meaning people that don't have the training to know differently. It fosters a sense of helplessness, leading to decreased motivation to seek solutions. It can be a self-fulfilling prophecy.

- **Limits Treatment Exploration:** It shuts down people's willingness to try new therapies, lifestyle changes, or seek out healthcare providers who focus on neuropathy.
- **Underestimates Possibilities:** While "cure" may not always be the outcome, significant improvement is possible for many. This includes:
  - Decreasing pain levels
  - Improving balance and mobility
  - Restoring some or all of your lost sensation
  - Slowing or reversing the progression of the disease.

Reality Check: Neuroplasticity and Hope

- **Neuroplasticity:** The nervous system has a remarkable ability to adapt and change – even in adulthood. Specialized therapies can stimulate this plasticity, prompting nerve repair and improving function.
- **Root-Cause Approach:** Many tools exist for finding and addressing the underlying drivers of your neuropathy (deficiencies, inflammation, etc.). Applied Kinesiology is one

of these amazing tools. Getting to the root is far more effective than just masking symptoms. This approach can lead to lasting improvements.

- **The Power of Self-Care:** Lifestyle changes that support nerve health can be incredibly impactful. This includes dietary adjustments, movement, and stress management. A daily nerve support routine is priceless.
- **Combined Therapies:** In my clinical experience, the greatest results come from a combination of personalized targeted home therapies, lifestyle optimization, in-office therapies and sometimes, medication (for immediate pain relief while deeper healing takes time).

The Takeaway: While neuropathy may pose challenges, it DOES NOT have to define your life. Refusing to accept the status quo empowers you to find solutions that optimize your function, reduce discomfort, and enhance your overall well-being. It's about mindset *-choosing to thrive* despite the limitations that neuropathy may bring.

By understanding these myths, you protect yourself from ineffective treatments, wasted time and money, and, most importantly, unnecessary suffering.

Knowledge and curiosity are your first defense against misinformation.

Real Stories Busting Myths: The Power of Informed Choices

The myths about neuropathy we've discussed don't just exist in theory – they have real consequences for people's lives. Here are a few stories showcasing how these misconceptions lead to delayed treatment, unnecessary suffering, and missed opportunities for improvement.

Story 1: The Misdiagnosed Diabetic

- **Patient:** Linda, a 65-year-old woman with a recent diabetes diagnosis. She developed numbness and tingling in her feet.
- **The Myth:** Her doctor assumed this was early diabetic neuropathy – a common assumption. No further testing was done.
- **The Reality:** Several years later, her symptoms worsened significantly. Seeking a second opinion, thorough testing revealed Linda had an autoimmune disease that attacked her stomach's ability to make the intrinsic factor needed for B12 absorption. This caused a severe vitamin B12 deficiency, a known cause of neuropathy.

- **The Consequence:** By the time the correct diagnosis was made, the nerve damage was more extensive. While the proper form of B12 supplementation helped, she could have regained more function with earlier intervention.

Story 2: The "Nerves Don't Heal" Nightmare

- **Patient:** Mark, a construction worker who injured his back in an accident. He had lingering leg pain and numbness post-surgery.
- **The Myth:** His surgeon told him, "Nerves don't grow back, you'll have to live with this." Mark felt hopeless and became depressed.
- **The Reality:** Years later, as his pain worsened, he sought help from a doctor who had extensive experience treating neuropathy and utilized Applied Kinesiology in his practice. Specialized therapies were prescribed and focused on re-establishing injured and over-stimulated nerve pathways, releasing nerve compression in the soft tissues and stimulating regeneration with red light and Pulsed electromagnetic field therapies. While some damage was permanent, he experienced significant improvement.

- **The Consequence:** The myth stole years of Mark's life. He became inactive due to pain, affecting his health and his once chipper spirit.

Story 3: Believing It's "Just Aging"

- **Patient:** Helen, a former dancer and vibrant 72-year-old, noticed increasing clumsiness and slight imbalance.
- **The Myth:** "What do you expect at your age?" she told herself, dismissing her symptoms.
- **The Reality:** A minor fall led to a fracture, sparking a thorough evaluation. Turns out, she had undiagnosed neuropathy due to a medication side effect.
- **The Consequence:** Her quality of life declined unnecessarily. With medication adjustment and personalized nerve rehab therapies, her balance improved, and she regained her confidence.

Protecting Yourself: Dangers of Misinformation and Finding Reliable Sources

In the age of the internet, anyone can publish "health" advice, making it hard to tell what's trustworthy and what's harmful. When it comes to neuropathy, misinformation can cost you time, money, and most critically, the chance for real improvement. Let's discuss the dangers and how to cut through the noise.

The Dangers of Misinformation

- **False Hope and Wasted Resources:** Unsubstantiated cures and miracle products prey on desperation. With a one-size-fits-all approach- they cost money and distract you from treatments with proven benefits.
- **Delayed Diagnosis and Treatment:** Believing myths (like neuropathy is only for diabetics or can't be improved) leads to missed opportunities for early intervention, when slowing the progression is often most feasible.
- **Harmful Choices:** Misinformation can lead people to try unproven remedies that worsen their condition, or to abandon conventional treatments they actually need.
- **Psychological Toll:** Constantly being disappointed by ineffective treatments breeds fear, resentment, humiliation and discouragement. This makes it harder to stay motivated and seek effective solutions.

How to Identify Reliable Information

- **Red Flags to Watch For:** Be skeptical of claims that sound too good to be true, like:
  - Instant cures or guaranteed results
  - Testimonials as the only "proof"
  - Secret formulas or blaming the medical establishment
- **Doctors with training** in effectively managing and improving neuropathy:
  - Seek out practitioners with advanced training or certifications in neuropathy, applied kinesiology, functional neurology, or related fields. They should have a proven track record of success in helping patients improve their condition, not just manage symptoms.
  - Ask about their approach. Do they offer a comprehensive assessment that looks beyond just medication? Do they consider lifestyle factors, nutrition, and other potential root causes?
  - Check for patient reviews. Online reviews and testimonials can offer insights into other patients' experiences with the practitioner.
- **Critical Thinking:** Ask questions like:

- Does the information you're finding about neuropathy treatment approaches align with what your doctor has explained?
  - Is the source trying to sell me something without any assessments or follow-up?
  - Are the benefits realistic or exaggerated?
- **Talk to Your Doctor:** If your Doctor is well-versed in natural holistic solutions, share any information you find with your healthcare team. They can help you determine its validity and whether it's relevant to your case. If they lack the experience, it's ok to find a second opinion from someone who is actually used to winning with your condition.

When it comes to your health, seeking reliable information is a powerful form of self-care. Empower yourself with knowledge, and you'll make better decisions on your path to healing.

Important Note: These stories don't mean everyone with neuropathy will have dramatic outcomes. But they illustrate why it's crucial to challenge assumptions, advocate for a thorough investigation, and pursue options beyond just symptom management.

Beyond the Basics: Common Misunderstood Aspects of Neuropathy

We've tackled major myths about neuropathy origins and treatment. But there are subtler misunderstandings that can also impact a patient's journey. Here's where the true complexity of this condition comes into focus.

Misconception #1: Neuropathy is just one disease.

Why It's Harmful

- **Oversimplified Treatment:** Assuming all neuropathy is the same leads to generic treatment approaches that may be ineffective or even counterproductive for certain types.
- **Frustration and Wasted Resources:** Patients get bounced between doctors or try therapies not suited for their type of neuropathy, leading to disappointment and wasted effort.
- **Missed Underlying Causes:** Treating a symptom without addressing the source of the nerve dysfunction is like putting a bandaid on a deep wound; it offers minimal, short-term relief at best.

Reality Check: Neuropathy Has Many Forms

Neuropathy is classified in numerous ways:

- Location:
  - Peripheral neuropathy – most common, affects extremities.
  - Autonomic neuropathy – impacts nerves controlling involuntary functions like digestion and heart rate.
  - Cranial neuropathy – affects nerves originating in the brain.
- Cause:
  - Diabetic neuropathy
  - Autoimmune neuropathy
  - Toxic neuropathy
  - Chemotherapy induced neuropathy
  - Idiopathic neuropathy (cause unknown)
  - Many more...
- Pattern of Damage:
  - Small fiber neuropathy – affects thin, unmyelinated nerve fibers. These are the pain nerves.
  - Large fiber neuropathy – affects thicker, myelinated nerves.
  - These can even have different symptom profiles.

The Importance of Specific Diagnosis

Knowing your type of neuropathy helps us:

- **Target the Root Cause:** Is it due to blood sugar dysregulation, an autoimmune process, something else or a combination of things? This determines the main treatment focus.
- **Choose Symptom-Specific Therapies:** Interventions, supplements, and therapies vary in effectiveness depending on the type of nerve damage.
- **Provide Prognosis Guidance:** Some neuropathies are more likely to improve than others. Understanding this helps set realistic expectations.

The Takeaway: "One neuropathy" doesn't exist. Working with a knowledgeable practitioner for thorough evaluation is crucial for personalized treatment that addresses the roots of YOUR nerve dysfunction.

Misconception #2: All neuropathy presents the same way.

Why It's Harmful

- **Delayed Diagnosis:** When people only expect "pins and needles," they may ignore or misunderstand other potential signs of neuropathy, hindering timely diagnosis and treatment.

- **Missed Treatment Opportunities:** Symptoms like bladder problems or dizziness might get written off as unrelated, leading to ineffective treatments that don't address the nerve dysfunction.

- **Unnecessary Worry:** Diverse symptoms that are actually due to neuropathy can cause confusion and anxiety as patients seek answers from the wrong specialists.

Reality Check: The Varied Faces of Neuropathy

Let's highlight the range of how neuropathy can manifest:

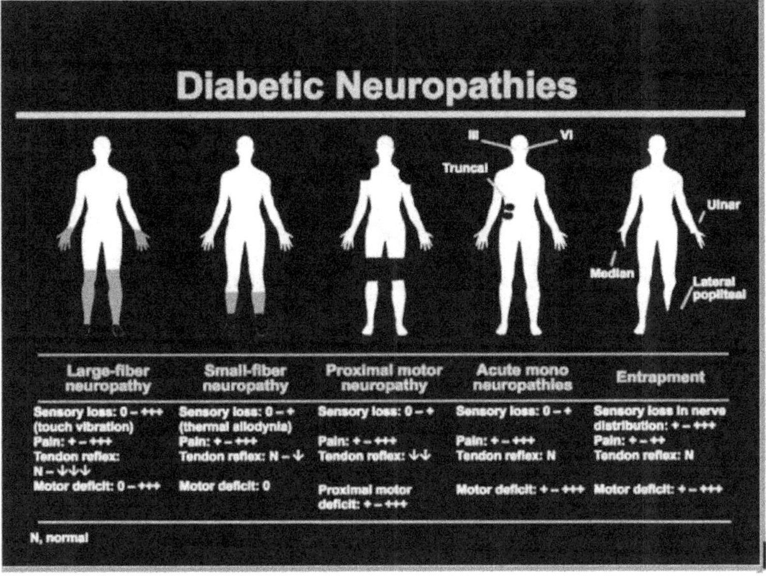

- Sensory Symptoms:
  - Burning, stabbing, or electric-shock sensations (often worse at night)
  - Extreme sensitivity to touch: even clothing or bed sheets can feel painful.
  - Numbness, loss of sensation, or temperature perception.
  - Difficulty feeling body position (can lead to falls).
- Motor Symptoms:
  - Muscle weakness: especially in hands/feet, causing clumsiness, dropping objects.
  - Muscle twitching or cramping.

- ○ Foot deformities (often in long-standing neuropathy).
- Autonomic Symptoms:
  - ○ Bladder issues: difficulty emptying, incontinence, frequent infections.
  - ○ Digestive problems: constipation, diarrhea, bloating.
  - ○ Blood pressure changes: dizziness upon standing, irregular heart rate.
  - ○ Sexual dysfunction, sweating abnormalities, and many others.

Why It Varies:

- Type of Nerves Affected: Sensory, motor, and autonomic nerves produce their own unique symptoms when damaged.
- Location: Nerves in different parts of the body produce different issues (leg nerves vs. nerves controlling digestion)
- Individual Variation: Even patients with the same type of neuropathy can have somewhat different symptom profiles.

The Takeaway: Neuropathy can masquerade as many other conditions. If you're experiencing unexplained, persistent symptoms – regardless of how unusual, discuss the possibility of neuropathy with your healthcare provider.

Misconception #3: Neuropathy only affects the limbs.

Why It's Harmful

- **Misdiagnosis and Mistreatment**: People with less common neuropathy locations may be misdiagnosed with entirely different conditions, leading to years of ineffective treatments.
- **Confounding Symptoms**: Not realizing symptoms are nerve-related causes unnecessary distress, as vague symptoms like fatigue or heart palpitations can lead to fear of serious diseases.
- **Delayed Intervention**: When nerves other than those in the extremities are involved, the urgency of getting a neuropathy diagnosis may be missed, hindering early intervention and optimal symptom resolution.

Reality Check: Neuropathy's Whole-Body Reach

- **Cranial Nerves**: These nerves originate in the brain and control facial expression, sensation, vision, hearing, taste, head rotation and more. Neuropathy can cause:

- Facial pain or numbness
- Neck, back and shoulder stiffness or weakness
- Vision changes (blurred vision, double vision)
- Hearing loss, tinnitus (ringing in the ears)
- Difficulty swallowing or speaking

- **Autonomic Nerves:** This system controls involuntary functions. Autonomic neuropathy can lead to:
  - Blood pressure problems (headaches,dizziness, lightheadedness)
  - Heart rhythm irregularities (too fast or too slow)
  - Digestive troubles (constipation, nausea, bloating)
  - Bladder dysfunction
  - Sexual difficulties
  - Sweating abnormalities (too much or too little)

- **Torso Nerves:** Nerve pain in the torso, back, or ribs can be mistaken for muscle pain, heartburn, or other issues.

Important Note: Not everyone with neuropathy will experience these symptoms. But their possibility is often overlooked, especially early on.

The Takeaway: Neuropathy can extend its reach far beyond the usual suspects. If you have persistent, unexplained symptoms in various parts of your body, mention the possibility of neuropathy to your doctor, even if you don't have classic numbness/tingling in your hands and feet. If your provider doesn't have extensive experience with neuropathy, consider getting a second opinion from a healthcare professional who has expertise in treating this condition.

Misconception #4: Neuropathy diagnosis is quick and easy.

Why It's Harmful:

- **Unreal Expectations:** This misconception sets patients up for frustration when a simple answer isn't forthcoming. This can lead to discouragement or prematurely giving up on seeking a diagnosis.
- **Oversimplified Treatment:** Getting a generic "neuropathy" diagnosis without root-cause identification means treatment is often guesswork with little chance of long-term success.

- **Missed Underlying Conditions:** Sometimes, neuropathy is the first sign of a serious but treatable medical condition. A thorough diagnostic process is essential to catch these.

Reality Check: The Detective Work of Neuropathy Diagnosis

Here's what might be involved in uncovering the "why" behind your neuropathy:

- **Detailed History and Exam:** Your doctor will ask about your symptoms, medical history, medications, family history, and exposure to potential toxins. This is the " L" in our LEGACY healing framework. We truly listen to see if your case is a match and how we can best help. Your history will help guide the "E" in our approach. Performing your Expert and Efficient physical/neurological exam - this is also key.
- **Blood, Urine or hair analysis Tests:** These go beyond the standard ones, often including:
  - Extensive vitamin panels (especially B vitamins)
  - Micronutrient panels (minerals and Fatty Acids)

- o Environmental Toxins and Heavy Metals (lead, mercury and others are deadly to the nerves)
  - o Markers of inflammation
  - o Autoimmune antibody testing. We often use the Array 5 panel from Cyrex Labs. This panel will screen 24 different body tissues for autoimmune attack. It can also show problems developing approximately 10 years before you would notice any symptoms.
  - o Specialized blood sugar and diabetes tests
- **Nerve Function Studies:**
  - o Electromyography (EMG): Measures electrical activity in muscles to assess nerve-muscle communication.
  - o Nerve Conduction Studies (NCS): Tests how fast signals travel along nerves. These help determine the type and pattern of damage.
  - o Physical Sensory Exam- there is no machine that can quantify what you feel. This is unique to you.

- **Imaging:**
  - For Neuropathy, standard MRIs are rarely helpful, BUT...if there is a disc problem or stenosis in the neck or lower back, this can complicate recovery. Make sure your provider is well versed in natural treatments for these conditions.
  - Specialized high-resolution ultrasound may be used to look for nerve compression or entrapment.
- **Genetic Testing:** In many cases, and especially in familial neuropathy, these tests can identify your specific inherited gene mutations that cause higher levels of chronic inflammation leading to nerve dysfunction. One mutation of note is endothelial NOS (eNOS) also known as nitric oxide synthase 3 (NOS3). This enzyme allows for the formation of nitric oxide- a vital nutrient that is used in many bodily functions.

Among other things, nitric oxide supports your body's normal blood flow mechanisms, brain protective processes, male and female healthy sexual responses, muscular strength processes, Human Growth Hormone activity and cholesterol-sulfate synthesis for heart energy. If you need this type of testing, be patient. It's not uncommon for lab results to take more than 3 months.

Important Note: Not everyone will need ALL of these tests. The diagnostic process is tailored to your unique presentation. Determining what tests to perform will be discussed with your doctor if it will change the course of treatment.

The Takeaway: Finding the source of your neuropathy requires patience and cooperation between you and your doctor. Thorough investigations increase the chances of finding targeted treatments that address the root of the problem, not just the symptoms.

Misconception #5: Neuropathy is always a chronic, progressive disease.

Why It's Harmful

- **Diminished Hope:** This misconception robs patients of the motivation to seek treatment or make lifestyle changes, fueling a sense of helplessness.
- **Missed Opportunities:** Even with chronic neuropathy, it's possible to slow or halt progression and significantly improve quality of life. Believing nothing can be done

squanders chances for improvement in quality of life.

- **Psychological Toll:** The fear of unrelenting decline takes an emotional toll, negatively impacting mood and overall well-being. This also tends to fast-forward the process because stress hormones further deplete an already tired system. The cycle goes around and around.

Reality Check: Neuropathy Comes in Various Forms

- **Temporary Neuropathy:**
  - Post-surgery: Nerves can be irritated during surgery, often improving over weeks or months as healing progresses. Commonly, a combination of proper nutrition, homeopathy, Pulsed Electromagnetic Field Therapy, nerve system balancing techniques and light therapy will shorten the healing time and speed recovery.
  - Vitamin deficiencies: Nerves need specific nutrients; correcting severe deficiencies (e.g., B12) can lead to significant improvement.
  - Acute Illnesses: Sometimes, infections or inflammatory conditions cause temporary

nerve dysfunction, resolving when the underlying issue is treated.

- **Stabilizable Neuropathy:**
  - Diabetic neuropathy: excellent blood sugar control is vital to slow progression, and therapies exist to improve nerve health- even reverse the diabetes that is driving the nerve damage in the first place.
  - Autoimmune neuropathy: Treating the underlying autoimmune disorder and quieting chronic inflammation is key to preventing further nerve damage.
- **Chronic, Progressive Neuropathy:** Even in cases without a cure, there's still much to gain:
  - Therapies can slow progression significantly.
  - Pain management is critical for quality of life.
  - Lifestyle changes support nerve health and overall well-being.

The Takeaway: While some neuropathies present more challenges than others, there is almost always something to be gained from thorough diagnosis, proactive treatment, and lifestyle optimization. Focus on what IS within your control, not just on what is not.

Neuropathy is a complex condition with many faces. Understanding these nuances protects you from one-size-fits-all treatments and helps you set realistic expectations for your healing journey.

The False Promise of Quick Fixes: Why They Fail in Neuropathy

Anyone suffering from neuropathy craves relief - it's understandable to be tempted by ads promising fast, effortless solutions. Sadly, these "quick fixes" rarely deliver. Let's explore why they fall short and how patients end up paying the price.

The Fallacy of Instant Cures

- **The Allure:** These "cures" play on desperation, using phrases like "secret formula," "reverse neuropathy overnight," or "what doctors don't want you to know."
- **The Reality:** Neuropathy is complex. A pill, cream, or device that supposedly works for everyone, regardless of the cause, is an impossible dream.
- **How They Exploit:** They often capitalize on these factors:
  - Lack of public understanding about neuropathy

- Limited options offered by some conventional doctors
- The placebo effect (people sometimes temporarily feel better just because they believe they should)
- **The Hidden Costs:**
  - Wasted money: The most expensive product is the one that doesn't work, regardless of price.
  - False hope: This undermines motivation for seeking truly effective solutions.
  - Delay: The time spent on ineffective cures delays finding treatments that might offer genuine help.

Stories of Failed Quick Fixes

- **The "Miracle Supplement" Trap:** Sarah, desperate to ease her burning feet, spent hundreds on a supplement advertised as "nerve regeneration in a bottle."No change occurred, leaving her stressed and discouraged.
- **The Gadget Gamble:** Mark tried an electrical stimulation device claiming to reverse neuropathy. While it provided a temporary tingling sensation, his underlying condition worsened.

- **The False Diagnosis Deception:** Desperate for answers, Linda visited a clinic advertising "groundbreaking neuropathy cures." They diagnosed her with a complex condition requiring a pricey, unproven treatment protocol. Later, a provider trained in Applied Kinesiology found a simple vitamin deficiency, confirmed with other standard diagnostics and it was easily addressed with supplements.

Remember: There is no substitute for a thorough diagnosis to identify the root cause of YOUR neuropathy. "One size fits all" solutions are destined to fail.

Beyond Symptom Relief: Choosing Sustainable Healing Over Short-Term Fixes

The desire for immediate relief from neuropathy pain is understandable. However, true healing requires a long-term perspective. Let's examine the difference between these approaches and why investing in a sustained path offers the best chance of lasting betterment.

Long-Term vs. Short-Term Thinking

- **Short-Term Focus: Symptom Suppression**
  - Examples: Pain medications, numbing creams, some off-the-shelf supplements.

- ○ Pros: May offer temporary relief in a crisis.
- ○ Cons: Doesn't fix the problem, often has side effects, can become less effective over time. Often a guessing game.
- **Long-Term Focus: Root-Cause Solutions & Sustainable Support**
  - ○ Examples: Treating nutritional deficiencies, gut health, blood sugar management, therapies to target nerve dysfunction, inflammation reduction, stress management, lifestyle modifications.
  - ○ Pros: Addresses the underlying cause of your neuropathy, offering the potential to significantly slow or halt its progression and improve your overall health. This, in turn, can reduce or eliminate the need for medication long-term.
  - ○ Cons: Requires investment of time and resources, patience, ongoing effort, and commitment to change.

Embracing Sustainable Healing

- **Why It's Worthwhile:** While not always fast or easy, this approach is your key to:
  - ○ Reduced pain, symptoms and improved function over time

- Less reliance on medication
- Minimizing likelihood of complications
- Enhanced overall well-being
- Improved quality of life
- **It's Not One or the Other:** There may be a role for short-term relief tactics (like medication) WHILE you pursue deeper healing.
- **Realistic Expectations:** Healing often isn't linear. Setbacks are normal. Celebrate small victories and maintain a focus on the bigger picture.
- **Partnership, Not a Magic Cure:** You play an active role in your success through diet, lifestyle adjustments, and adherence to therapy. Your healthcare team provides guidance and support.

Sustainable healing means investing in yourself, both physically and mentally. While instant cures are appealing, choosing strategies that address the root of your neuropathy and promote overall health is the path toward lasting improvements in your quality of life.

Your Roadmap to Lasting Relief: Strategies for Sustainable Healing

Let's dive into specific examples of long-term neuropathy strategies that target root causes and support overall nerve health. Note: These are not universally applicable to everyone – they highlight the range of approaches that might be part of a personalized treatment plan.

Addressing Specific Root Causes:

- **Diabetic Neuropathy:**
    - Intensive blood sugar management (diet, fasting, medication, monitoring)
    - Therapies for circulation improvement (e.g., specialized light therapy, Physical Vascular Therapy etc.)
    - Supplements to support nerve health (R-alpha-lipoic acid, benfotiamine , berberine, Lion's mane and others– discuss with your doctor)
- **Nutritional Deficiencies:**
    - Replenishing specific vitamins/minerals crucial for nerve function (especially magnesium, B vitamins and vitamin D) via diet and targeted supplementation.
    - Addressing underlying gut issues that may impair absorption for many people. Foods high in histamine and oxalates may contribute to pain. Additionally, dysbiosis from subclinical low level gut infections-

yeast, some bacteria, funguses and molds often cause significant exacerbation.

- **Autoimmune Neuropathy:**
  - You must identify what's driving your immune system to attack your body- food reactions, infections like chronic viruses or tick-borne diseases, molds etc. and heavy metals can play a causative role.
  - Glutathione- the body's master antioxidant
  - Immune-suppressing medication (if appropriate for your specific diagnosis)
  - Anti-inflammatory diet and lifestyle interventions
  - Therapies tailored to the specific autoimmune condition affecting your nerves.
- **Toxic Neuropathy:**
  - Identifying and eliminating the toxin (e.g., heavy metals, certain medications or chemotherapy agents)
  - Support for detoxification (under medical guidance)
  - Therapies to support nerve regeneration.

Nerve-Supportive Therapies (May be beneficial across various neuropathy types):

- **Specialized Neuro-Physical Therapy:** To improve balance, gait, and muscle strength, and address nerve entrapment issues.
- **Regenerative Therapies:** Examples include certain forms of light therapy, digital electro-therapeurtic stimulation, Pulsed Electromagnetic Field Therapy, Physical vascular therapy, Tissue Regeneration Therpy and others undergoing research.
- **Mind-Body Interventions:** Neuro-Emotional Technique, Stress reduction techniques, mindfulness, relaxation training, singing with a group of people – calming the nervous system is key.

Lifestyle Modifications Supporting Long-Term Healing:

- **Anti-Inflammatory Diet:** Rich in fruits, vegetables, healthy fats, limiting processed foods. This reduces a major driver of nerve damage.
- **Regular Movement:** Safe, doctor-approved exercise improves circulation, supports nerve health, and boosts mood.
- **Sleep Optimization:** Essential for repair and reducing nerve pain sensitivity.

- **Stress Management:** Chronic stress worsens neuropathy. Tools like deep breathing, meditation, and enjoyable activities are crucial.

Important Disclaimer: This list is NOT a substitute for consulting a knowledgeable healthcare provider. Strategies need to be individualized based on your diagnosis, health history, and current needs. Call us at 717-285-0001 or visit our website, getwellandstaywell. com/contact, to schedule an appointment. This is an opportunity to discuss your health concerns and explore potential treatment options, but does not guarantee specific results. The LEGACY program may not be suitable for everyone.

The Power of Lifestyle: Your Secret Weapon Against Neuropathy

While medications and therapies have their place, true neuropathy management extends far beyond the doctor's office. Your daily habits, diet, and how you manage stress play a crucial role in either fueling nerve dysfunction or creating an environment where healing can occur. Let's explore the key lifestyle factors that matter.

Lifestyle Factors in Neuropathy

Nutrition: The Nerve Nourishment Factor

Your nerves need a steady supply of specific vitamins, minerals, and antioxidants to function properly and protect themselves from damage. A diet lacking in nutrient-rich whole foods and filled with processed junk fuels inflammation, a major driver of neuropathy. Conversely, an anti-inflammatory diet abundant in fruits, vegetables, healthy fats, and lean protein can be powerfully healing.

Blood Sugar Dysregulation: A Hidden Driver

Uncontrolled blood sugar levels, whether you have full-blown diabetes or are just beginning with insulin resistance, wreak havoc on nerves. Stabilizing blood sugar is imperative for preventing neuropathy or slowing its progression. This involves diet but may also require supplements and/or medication for some individuals.

Movement is Medicine

The right kind, intensity and duration of exercise improves circulation, essential for bringing oxygen and nutrients to damaged nerves. It also helps manage blood sugar, reduces stress and stimulates energy production. Finding safe, enjoyable ways to move your body regularly can make a significant difference in your neuropathy symptoms and overall health. This is where a professional applied kinesiologist can really be of assistance. Trained in how the brain, nerves and muscles coordinate movement, the applied kinesiologist can find and correct aberrant gait patterns and faulty biomechanics that limit healthy movement. When you can't move properly, it robs the brain of the vital input it needs to adapt to its environment. Dysfunction is the precursor to dis-ease.

The Stress-Nerve Connection

Traumatic stress and chronic stress keep your nervous system in a constant state of survival. This will manifest in at least one of three responses to the perceived threat. You can kick into overdrive to "fight", retreat or run to "flee", or "freeze" like a deer in the headlights. This response is involuntary. In this state, you are most concerned with keeping the vital organs going - not in healing mode. Over time, this can lead to "burnout" and /or "numbing"- one of the late stages of neuropathy. Stress management techniques like deep diaphragmatic breathing, mindfulness, spending time in nature, or therapies like acupuncture, massage, or simply giving and receiving hugs can offer a huge boost to your healing journey. One of the most researched and successful treatments for the stress-nerve connection is Neuro Emotional Technique or NET. NET helps individuals identify and modify negative thought patterns that can develop behaviors that contribute to stress and pain perception. It balances the neurophysiology in the brain- resetting the stress physiology. This neutralizes the effects of stressful emotional triggers thereby reducing its impact on the nervous system and promoting healing.

The Importance of Restorative Sleep

Sleep deprivation ramps up pain and makes it harder to cope with neuropathy. Prioritizing sleep habits and your sleep environment supports nerve repair and reduces your sensitivity to discomfort.

Mattress Tips:

- So how old is your mattress? If it's over a decade it's probably time to upgrade.
- Look for support and comfort. Avoid spring coils that can add pressure points and restrict blood flow. Avoid memory foam that traps heat and can contribute to body fluid stagnation.
- Consider air cell technology that removes pressure points regardless of sleep position. I personally use Natural Form mattresses and recommend them to my patients naturalform.com.

Examples of Lifestyle Impact

While more research is always welcome, here's a glimpse at how lifestyle changes can have measurable effects:

- **Reduced Pain:** Diet changes, stress management, and targeted exercise are shown to decrease neuropathy pain and improve quality of life.
- **Improved Function:** Better nutrition, building strength, and working on balance with specialized brain and muscle therapy may translate to better mobility, fewer falls, and increased independence.
- **Need for Less Medication:** As healing progresses with lifestyle optimization, some patients can eliminate their reliance on pain medication and its side effects.

Lifestyle isn't an afterthought in neuropathy treatment – it's a cornerstone of your healing journey. Small, consistent changes over time can create profound effects on your pain levels, function, and quality of life. I've seen these positive results happen consistently and repeatedly in my own practice and with colleagues around the country and the globe.

Transform Your Health, Transform Your Life: The Benefits of Lifestyle Change in Neuropathy

Often, when we think of medical treatments, we imagine medications or procedures. However, with neuropathy, some of the most powerful tools for healing are in your hands – the choices you make every day. Let's explore the multifaceted ways lifestyle shifts can enhance your well-being.

Benefits of Lifestyle Adjustments

- **Pain Reduction and Improved Function:** Lifestyle changes address underlying drivers of neuropathy pain, like inflammation and blood sugar dysregulation, leading to gradual, sustainable improvement in pain, numbness, and physical function.
- **Reduced Medication Reliance:** When lifestyle supports healing, the need for pain medication often lessens, minimizing side effects and improving overall health.
- **Slowed Progression:** In many types of neuropathy, lifestyle optimization is key to slowing the disease process, preventing further nerve damage and minimizing complications.
- **Enhanced Overall Health:** The changes that benefit your nerves also benefit your heart,

metabolism, and immune system. You reduce risk for other chronic illnesses, improving vitality for years to come.

- **Mental and Emotional Well-being**: Chronic pain takes a mental toll. As physical symptoms improve, so do mood and anxiety. Moreover, the act of taking healthy steps is empowering, boosting your confidence.

Lifestyle Change Recommendations (Focus Areas)

- **Diet**: Shift towards an anti-inflammatory diet rich in organic and non-GMO:
  - Fruits & Vegetables: Packed with antioxidants and nerve-healthy nutrients.
  - Healthy Fats: Avocados, nuts, oily fish (great for reducing inflammation)
  - Lean Protein: Important for nerve and muscle health.Research shows that humans need between 1.2-2.0 grams per kilogram of body weight. This can help with maintaining muscle mass and weight loss.
  - Emphasis on whole, unprocessed foods, avoiding artificial sweeteners, sugar (white, brown, raw, coconut, turbinado etc.) and refined carbs is a must

- **Movement:**
  - Find enjoyable activities that fit your abilities. Walking, swimming, chair exercises – consistency is key.
  - Talk to your doctor or a physical therapist for guidance if needed.
- **Sleep:**
  - Consistent sleep/wake times, even on weekends.
  - Relaxing bedtime routine, dark and quiet sleep environment.
  - Address sleep issues like apnea with your doctor.
- **Stress Management:**
  - Mind-body practices: First Aid Stress Tool (www.firstaidstresstool.com) Heart Math exercises, deep breathing, meditation, yoga etc.
  - Enjoyable hobbies and activities that bring you pleasure. Trying new things and experiences - the brain enjoys novelty.
  - Seek counseling and treatment from a certified Neuro Emotional Technique practitioner before stress gets overwhelming. If you're dealing with a chronic health challenge like neuropathy,

then the odds are good that you've had some kind of mental/ emotional stress in your life. Even from childhood, many are exposed to the death of a loved one, physical, verbal or sexual abuse. In fact, according to rainn.org, every 68 seconds an American is sexually assaulted- every 9 minutes that victim is a child. Nationally, 50% of marriages end in divorce. In my clinical experience, sometimes, the physical pain and numbing that people experience with neuropathy is a physical manifestation of the abuse or traumatic emotional pain and subsequent numbing of that emotional pain.

Important Note: Lifestyle changes work best in conjunction with necessary treatments and the often multi-faceted root-cause identification. Talk to us about how to safely integrate them into your plan.

The Takeaway: Empower yourself! While these changes require effort, the rewards are transformative. By committing to a healthier lifestyle, you invest in a future with reduced pain, increased function, and the ability to live your life to the fullest.

Feeling Again: Nancy's LEGACY of Renewed Hope

"When I started the LEGACY program, I had 47% loss of feeling in my right foot and 43% in my left. My shoulder had limited range of motion, and I woke up with headaches every morning.

Now, just a few months later, I've regained almost half the feeling in my feet! I can feel textures again, and I can walk a mile and a half – something I couldn't do for a long time. Even my shoulder has improved, and those morning headaches are gone.

It takes dedication, but it's worth it. I've even recommended LEGACY to others who are suffering. Don't let anyone tell you there's no hope for neuropathy – I'm living proof that healing is possible!"

** Every patient's journey is unique. This testimonial does not guarantee similar results for others.*

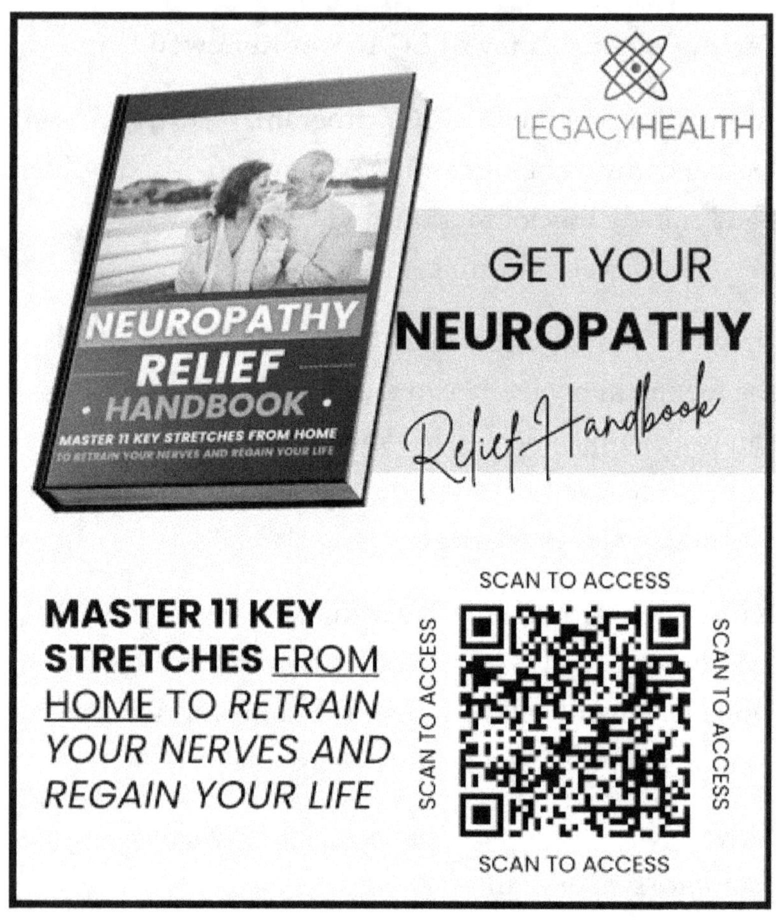

Unlock Your Path to Neuropathy Relief Now: Call 717-285-0001 to Speak With a Skilled Neuropathy Professional Today!

4

BLOOD SUGAR SECRETS: UNLOCKING THE KEY TO NEUROPATHY PREVENTION

The American Diet Decimates Blood Sugar

Whether you have diabetic neuropathy or not, proper blood sugar balance is a necessity for proper nerve health. The food landscape we navigate daily is packed with sugary drinks, processed snacks, and refined carbohydrates. While these might offer short-term satisfaction, they destroy our blood sugar control, setting the stage for a host of health problems, including peripheral neuropathy.

The Pivotal Role of Balanced Blood Sugar

Our nerves, like every other cell in our body, require a steady supply of energy in the form of glucose (sugar) from our bloodstream. However, too much glucose is toxic. Precisely balanced blood sugar levels are essential for:

- **Optimal Nerve Function:** Nerves need the right amount of glucose for energy, but excesses cause direct damage.
- **Reducing Inflammation:** Chronically high blood sugar drives inflammation, a major factor in nerve damage.
- **Healthy Blood Flow:** Spikes and crashes in blood sugar impair circulation, reducing oxygen and nutrient delivery to nerves, especially in the extremities.
- **Body Mechanics:** Blood sugar imbalances inhibit arm and leg muscles that control gait, maintain balance and mobility.

In this chapter, we'll uncover how the typical American diet sabotages blood sugar control and explore the direct consequences this has on your nerves. Understanding this connection is the first step towards protecting your health and preventing the potential devastation of neuropathy.

The Sweet Assault: How the American Diet Causes Blood Sugar Imbalance

From sugary cereals to oversized sodas and refined-carb snacks, the American food landscape is built upon convenience rather than true nourishment. While these foods might provide immediate gratification, they send our blood sugar on a rollercoaster ride, with disastrous long-term effects on our nerves and overall health.

Overview of the Typical American Diet's Impact on Blood Sugar

- **Refined Carbohydrate Overload:** Breads, cakes, cookies, pastas, pastries, sugary snacks and drinks, and processed foods are quickly broken down into glucose, overwhelming the body's ability to process it efficiently, leading to spikes in blood sugar.
- **Sugar Saturation:** Added sugars lurk everywhere - in beverages, sauces, condiments, dressings, and even seemingly "healthy" yogurt and protein bars. These add to the overall sugar burden, triggering rapid blood sugar increases.
- **Lack of Fiber:** Most processed foods are devoid of fiber, which is crucial for slowing the absorption of sugar into the bloodstream. Without fiber, blood sugar levels rise rapidly.
- **Inflammatory Fats:** The abundance of unhealthy fats (trans fats, seed oils, excessive

saturated fats) in processed foods contributes to inflammation, which worsens the body's ability to manage blood sugar.

The typical American dietary pattern creates a perfect storm of blood sugar chaos, characterized by sharp spikes followed by energy crashes, leaving us craving more of the very foods that perpetuate the problem.

The Blood Sugar Saboteurs: Refined Carbs, Sugars, and Processed Foods

While essential in their whole-food forms, carbohydrates, and sugars become detrimental to health when heavily refined and processed. Let's break down why these ubiquitous "dietary staples" are such a threat to blood sugar balance and, ultimately, nerve health.

The Refined Carbohydrate Trap

- **Stripped of Their Value:** Foods like bread, white rice, corn and many cereals have been stripped of fiber and nutrients. They are essentially pure starch, rapidly converted into glucose in the body.
- **Blood Sugar Surges:** These foods cause sharp spikes in blood sugar, putting stress on the system and increasing insulin output. Over

time, this impairs the body's ability to manage blood sugar.

- **The Energy Rollercoaster:** The rapid spike is followed by a crash as insulin overcompensates. This leads to cravings, and increased hunger, and perpetuates blood sugar instability. This starts as reactive hypoglycemia and eventually exhausts the pancreas' ability to make insulin and full blown diabetes follows.

The Hidden Sweetness: Added Sugars

- **Not Just the Sugar Bowl:** Added sugars are everywhere - sodas, candy, juices, flavored yogurts, and even pasta sauces. They contribute massively to our total sugar intake.
- **More Than Just Empty Calories:** Added sugars trigger the same sharp blood sugar fluctuations as refined carbs, driving inflammation, and increasing neuropathy risk.
- **The Illusion of Health:** Often disguised as "natural" sweeteners (agave, coconut sugar, turbinado, raw, maple syrup, etc.), they still have the same detrimental effects on blood sugar.

Processed Foods - A Perfect Storm

- **Combined Assault:** Most processed foods are a combination of refined carbs, added sugars, unhealthy fats, and minimal nutritional value. They're designed for addictive appeal, not health.
- **Inflammation Fuel:** The ingredients and processing techniques used in these foods promote chronic inflammation – a key player in nerve damage and impaired blood sugar control.

While delicious and seemingly unavoidable, the heavy reliance on refined carbs, added sugars, and processed foods in the standard American diet sets the stage for blood sugar dysfunction, creating a breeding ground for neuropathy and other chronic illnesses.

Blood Sugar Spikes: The Silent Assault on Your Nerves

Beyond the fatigue, cravings, and mood swings associated with blood sugar swings, each spike has deceptively dangerous effects that accumulate over time. Understanding the immediate impact on our nerves highlights the urgency of prioritizing blood sugar stability for neuropathy prevention.

The Instant Assault

- **Glucose Surge:** After a carb-heavy or sugary meal, blood sugar levels rise rapidly. This overwhelms the system and creates a state of excess glucose in the bloodstream.
- **Oxidative Stress Explosion:** High glucose levels trigger a cascade of oxidative stress, which essentially causes cell damage by these harmful inflammatory molecules called free radicals. Nerves are especially vulnerable to this type of damage.
- **Inflammation Ignition:** Blood sugar swings promote a state of chronic inflammation throughout the body. This inflammation directly injures nerves and worsens overall health.

The Cycle of Nerve Damage

- **Nerve Cell Starvation:** While blood sugar is high, cells struggle to get the glucose for energy due to insulin dysfunction. It's a paradox of too much fuel, yet cellular starvation.
- **Direct Toxicity:** Excess glucose is directly toxic to the delicate structures within nerves, causing dysfunction and potentially irreversible damage.

- **Reduced Circulation:** Blood sugar extremes impair small blood vessel health. This reduces oxygen and nutrients to the nerves, especially in the extremities (hands, feet and brain).

Each time we indulge in foods that send our blood sugar soaring, it's not just a temporary alert. It contributes to the ongoing silent damage to our nerves. Over the years, this damage manifests as the pain, numbness, and complications of neuropathy.

Diet-Driven Destruction: Inflammation, Oxidative Stress, and Neuropathy

The typical American diet, loaded with refined carbohydrates, unhealthy fats, and added sugars, isn't just about excess calories. It creates a state of low-grade, chronic inflammation and oxidative stress throughout the body. Nerves are highly susceptible to this kind of damage, paving the way for neuropathy.

Inflammation: The Fire Within

- **Diet's Inflammatory Impact:** Processed foods, Genetically modified, pesticide soaked "conventionally grown" foods, excess sugar, and unhealthy fats directly trigger inflammatory cascades in the body.

- **Nerve Onslaught:** This inflammation directly attacks nerves. It may manifest as burning pain, hypersensitivity, and an increased risk of nerve fiber damage.
- **Self-Perpetuating Cycle:** Damaged nerves themselves release inflammatory signals, exacerbating the problem.

Oxidative Stress: Cellular Rusting

- **Reactive Oxygen Species (ROS):** High blood sugar, toxins, and an inflammatory diet lead to excess production of ROS, which is like cellular "rust," causing damage to DNA, proteins, and cell membranes.
- **Nerves Under Attack:** Nerve cells are particularly vulnerable to oxidative stress due to their high metabolic activity and structure.
- **The Consequences:** Oxidative stress damages nerve fibers, impairs nerve signal transmission, and makes nerves more susceptible to other forms of injury. Like all rusty things, they break down much quicker.

The chronic inflammation and oxidative stress triggered by a poor diet aren't just abstract concepts – they are potent forces that directly contribute to nerve dysfunction and increase the likelihood of developing neuropathy. Every dietary choice is either supporting a healthy internal environment, or contributing to the breakdown of tissues – including the nerves.

The Dietary Disaster: How It Sets the Stage for Neuropathy

By now, the picture is becoming alarmingly clear. The typical American diet isn't just about excess calories; it's a recipe for metabolic dysfunction and a direct pathway to nerve damage. Let's summarize the major ways it sets the stage for neuropathy:

1. **Relentless Blood Sugar Spikes & Crashes:** Heavy reliance on refined carbohydrates, added sugars, and processed foods leads to constant blood sugar instability, stressing the entire system, promoting insulin resistance, and directly damaging nerves.

2. **Chronic Inflammation:** This diet creates a constant state of low-grade inflammation throughout the body, directly harming nerves, impairing blood flow, and making neuropathy more likely.

3. **Oxidative Stress Overload:** Excess sugar and unhealthy fats trigger the overproduction of harmful molecules (ROS), which damage nerve cells and their delicate structures.

4. Nutritional Deficiencies: Processed foods are devoid of the vitamins and minerals crucial for nerve health (especially B vitamins and magnesium).They also require the use of these crucial nutrients to metabolize and promote excretion, further depleting the body. They are "anti-nutrients". This leaves nerves even more vulnerable to damage.

5. Gut Health Disruption: The lack of fiber and the presence of inflammatory and toxic compounds in the diet disrupt gut bacteria balance. Other microbes like viruses, funguses, molds and parasites can get a strong foothold. Poor gut health is connected to worsened blood sugar control and increased inflammation – both neuropathy risk factors.

The Takeaway: It's not any one food that's the culprit, but the overall pattern. The standard American diet bombards our bodies with triggers that lead to blood sugar chaos, inflammation, oxidative stress, and ultimately nerve damage. Years of this dietary disaster create a breeding ground for neuropathy.

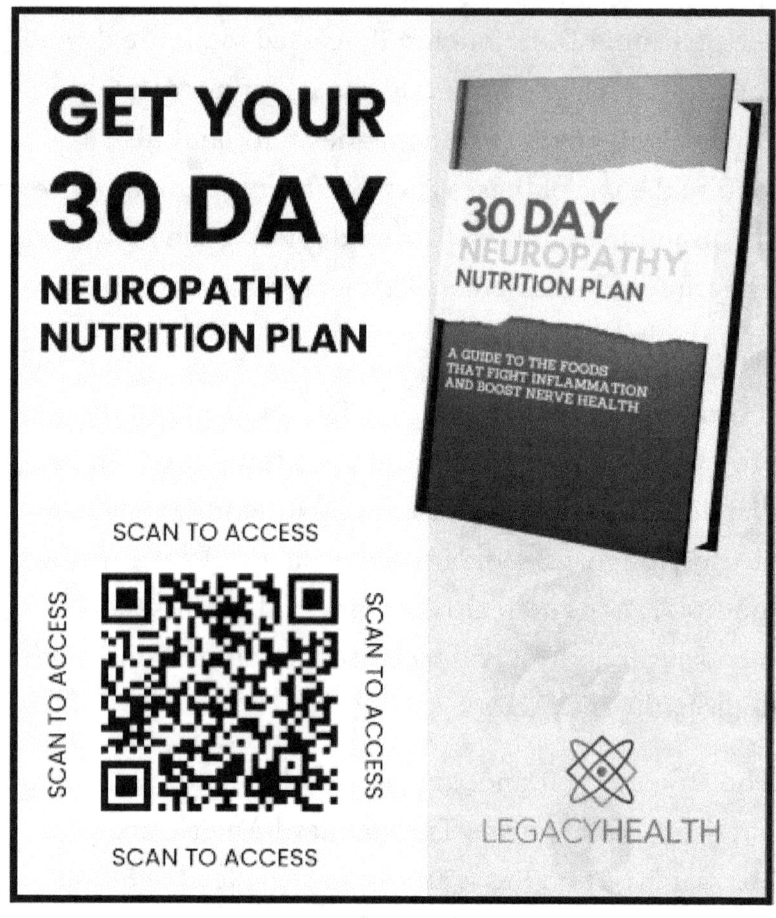

Insulin, Glucagon, and the Blood Sugar Tango (and How to Keep Them Dancing)

Maintaining stable blood sugar levels is a delicate dance, orchestrated primarily by two key hormones: insulin and glucagon. Understanding their roles is essential for grasping how imbalances contribute to neuropathy. Let's focus on insulin first, the hormone most often associated with blood sugar issues.

The Indispensable Role of Insulin

Think of insulin as your body's "sugar usher." After a meal, when blood sugar rises, the pancreas releases insulin. Here's its multifaceted job:

- **Cell Door Unlocker:** Insulin signals cells throughout your body (primarily muscle and liver cells) to open "doors" and allow glucose to enter for energy or storage.
- **Storage Activator:** Insulin instructs the liver to take in excess glucose and store it as glycogen, ensuring a steady fuel supply between meals.
- **Fat Storage Promoter:** When energy needs are met, insulin also facilitates the storage of excess glucose as fat.This can cause fatty liver disease and unhealthy levels of visceral and abdominal fat

Insulin, Glucose Uptake, and Neuropathy

It's easy to blame insulin when blood sugar is high, but without it, our cells would starve! Here's the link to neuropathy:

- **Cellular "Hunger" in Neuropathy:** When cells become resistant to insulin's message (more on this later), they fail to get the glucose they need, even if blood levels are high. This impairs nerve cell function and health.
- **Direct Toxicity:** In states of chronically elevated blood sugar, nerves are exposed to damaging levels of glucose, leading to structural damage.
- **Inflammation Trigger:** High insulin levels themselves (a sign of insulin resistance) promote inflammation, which injures nerves.

Insulin plays a vital role in regulating blood sugar after we eat. However, problems arise when our cells become resistant to its effects or when insulin production falters – these scenarios are primary drivers of neuropathy development.

The Blood Sugar Seesaw: Insulin, Glucagon, and Neuropathy Protection

While insulin gets most of the attention, glucagon plays an equally important role in maintaining healthy blood sugar levels. Think of it as the accelerator to insulin's brake. Let's see how glucagon works and why the balance between the two is so crucial.

Glucagon: The Blood Sugar Stabilizer

- **Glucagon's Job:** When blood sugar levels drop (between meals, after exercise), the pancreas releases glucagon. It primarily targets the liver, triggering these actions:
    - **Release of Stored Glucose:** Glucagon signals the liver to break down glycogen and release glucose back into the bloodstream, preventing blood sugar from going too low.
    - **New Glucose Production:** It can even stimulate the production of new glucose, ensuring a steady supply.
- **Relevance to Neuropathy:** Glucagon helps protect nerves by preventing hypoglycemic episodes (very low blood sugar), which can directly damage nerves and worsen symptoms in those who already have neuropathy.

The Insulin-Glucagon Balance & Neuropathy Prevention

Our bodies are designed for fluctuations in blood sugar, but within a narrow range. Here's how the insulin-glucagon teamwork keeps things stable (when everything's working correctly):

- **Post-Meal Rise Controlled:** Insulin goes to work to bring blood sugar down after eating, preventing excessive spikes.
- **Glucose Supply Maintained:** As levels start to dip, glucagon acts as a safety net, ensuring enough glucose for brain and nerve function.
- **Constant Adjustment:** Throughout the day, this fine-tuned system responds to meals, activity, and even stress levels, making sure blood sugar stays in a safe zone.

When the Balance Breaks Down

Developing chronic conditions like insulin resistance and diabetes disrupt this delicate harmony. It can lead to blood sugar levels that swing wildly or remain chronically high – both scenarios create a toxic environment for our nerves.

The Takeaway: Optimal nerve health relies on both insulin and counter-regulatory hormones of glucagon (with growth hormone, epinephrine and cortisol) working effectively. A disrupted blood sugar control system is a major contributor to the development of neuropathy.

Insulin Resistance: The Silent Path to Neuropathy

Insulin resistance doesn't happen overnight. It tends to develop gradually, often with vague symptoms easily dismissed as simply "getting older." However, recognizing the early signs provides an opportunity to reverse course and protect your nerves.

Early Warning Signs: When Cells Stop Listening

1. **Cellular Resistance to Insulin:** The root of the problem is when cells throughout the body become less responsive to insulin's signal. Think of it as the volume being turned down – cells don't get enough glucose, even as blood sugar levels creep higher. Here's where neuropathy enters the picture:
   - Nerve "Hunger": Nerve cells, like all cells, require steady glucose for optimal function. Insufficient supply due to insulin resistance contributes to dysfunction and symptoms like tingling and subtle numbness.
   - Early Blood Vessel Damage: Elevated blood sugar, even at modest levels, starts to damage small blood vessels that nourish nerves.
2. **Elevated Post-Meal Blood Sugar:** Here's how this ties in:

- ○ The "Lag Time": Cells are slow to take in glucose due to insulin resistance. This means blood sugar stays higher for longer after meals.
- ○ Damage in Progress: Even these occasional spikes lead to oxidative stress and inflammation, injuring nerves over time. Note: Fasting blood sugar may still look normal in the early stages! It can be helpful to measure a postprandial blood sugar level 1 hour after eating. Optimal levels should be below 140.

3. What are some of the warning signs of insulin resistance?

- Increased thirst.
- Frequent urination (peeing).
- Increased hunger.
- Blurred vision.
- Headaches.
- Vaginal and skin infections.
- Slow-healing cuts and sores.
- Unexplained shoulder problems, mid and lower back pain or ankle weakness and arch problems.

Key Points to Emphasize

- Subtlety is Deceiving: Early insulin resistance signs might be fatigue, increased hunger/cravings, moderately elevated blood pressure above 130/80, or difficulty losing weight... not necessarily classic neuropathy symptoms.
- Prevention Window: This is NOT an inevitable path. Lifestyle changes made early on can reverse insulin resistance and protect your nerves.
- Professional Applied Kinesiologists are trained to find the muscle imbalance patterns associated with insulin resistance and blood sugar handling problems and support the underlying causes- physical, chemical and emotional.

Even before full-blown diabetes is diagnosed, blood sugar dysregulation silently damages nerves. Understanding these initial stages is key for prevention, emphasizing the need to look beyond fasting blood sugar tests alone. Consider measuring hemoglobin A1C, fasting insulin, and NMR LipoProfile® With Insulin Resistance Markers.

Moderate Insulin Resistance: The Danger Zone for Neuropathy

As insulin resistance worsens, cells become stubbornly resistant to insulin's message. The pancreas tries to compensate by pumping out even more insulin, but the blood sugar situation spirals out of control. This stage sets the stage for serious health issues, including neuropathy.

Impaired Glucose Tolerance: A Warning Sign

- What It Means: Impaired glucose tolerance, often called "prediabetes," means blood sugar levels are consistently higher than normal after meals, BUT not high enough for a diabetes diagnosis yet.
- The Nerves Suffer: Even in this "pre" stage, nerves are exposed to damaging levels of glucose. Structural damage progresses, potentially leading to worsening neuropathy symptoms.
- Inflammation Escalates: As discussed above, chronically elevated blood sugar means constant inflammation, a major driver of nerve dysfunction and pain.
- Impaired mobility: blood sugar problems affect muscles that support the shoulder, knee, ankle,

neck and back. Chronic muscle tone imbalance (over-facilitation or inhibition) promotes accelerated joint wear and tear. Decreased mobility, joint pain and stiffness symptoms can develop or progressively get worse. Fall risk is also heightened from injured or weakened tissues.

- Visceral Fat: Increased abdominal fat (the deep belly fat) is strongly linked to insulin resistance. This type of fat releases inflammatory compounds that fast-forward the problem.
- Metabolic Syndrome: This cluster of risk factors often accompanies moderate insulin resistance and dramatically increases neuropathy risk. Criteria include:
  - Large waistline
  - High blood pressure
  - High triglycerides (blood fats)
  - Low HDL ("good" cholesterol)
- The Dire Consequences: Metabolic syndrome significantly accelerates blood vessel damage, including those supplying nerves, worsening neuropathy and increasing risk for cardiovascular complications.

Moderate insulin resistance means the body is actively fighting a losing battle against blood sugar dysregulation. This is a critical point – neuropathy is a serious concern, but lifestyle changes can significantly improve your health and may help prevent further nerve damage.

Severe Insulin Resistance: Neuropathy's Perfect Storm

Severe insulin resistance means the body's blood sugar control system is severely compromised. Cells remain unresponsive, creating chronically high blood sugar. Meanwhile, the pancreas, struggling to keep up, starts to falter. This combination is devastating for the nerves.

Chronic High Blood Sugar: Nerve Cell Sabotage

- The Constant bombardment: Now, blood sugar isn't just spiking after meals – it's persistently elevated. Nerves are bathed in damaging glucose.
- Advanced Damage: Mechanisms like oxidative stress, inflammation, and direct glucose toxicity accelerate, leading to structural changes in nerve fibers.
- Increased Complications: Severe neuropathy progresses, with worsening pain, numbness, potential for infections, and impaired wound healing.

Beta-Cell Exhaustion: Losing Critical Function

- The Pancreas Falters: Beta cells in the pancreas, responsible for making insulin, become overworked and damaged in severe insulin resistance.
- Insulin Production Plummets: Even if blood sugar is high, the body becomes unable to make enough insulin to counteract it. This often marks the progression to type 2 diabetes.
- Losing a Safeguard: While insulin gets a bad rap, it has some protective effects for nerves. In its absence, nerve damage progresses more rapidly.

Severe insulin resistance creates an environment where neuropathy flourishes. While blood sugar control remains vital even at this stage to slow progression, nerve damage has likely become significant and less reversible. This underscores the importance of NOT allowing it to reach this point.

Overworked Insulin: How a "Good Thing" Turns Harmful for Nerves

In the early stages of insulin resistance, the body tries to compensate for cells not responding to insulin by producing more and more of the hormone. This relentless overproduction of insulin itself has negative consequences, including for your nerves.

Recognizing Insulin Fatigue

- Not Just About Blood Sugar: While blood sugar may still look "controlled," high insulin levels (hyperinsulinemia) are a sign the system is overburdened.
- Key Consequences for Nerves:
  - **Inflammation:** High insulin directly promotes inflammation, worsening the environment for nerves.
  - **Weight Gain:** Excess insulin drives fat storage, worsening insulin resistance – a vicious cycle.
  - **Direct Nerve Effects:** Some research suggests excessive insulin over long periods might have damaging effects on nerves[1].

Prolonged High Insulin and Neuropathy Risk

- **Increased Risk:** Studies show that even without full-blown diabetes, high insulin levels are associated with an increased risk of neuropathy[1].

- **Metabolic Damage:** Hyperinsulinemia contributes to a cascade of issues like high blood pressure, and dyslipidemia (unhealthy cholesterol profile), all accelerating vascular damage that impairs nerve health.
- **Often Silent:** High insulin can exist for years before blood sugars become truly abnormal, causing hidden damage during this time.

We tend to focus on high blood sugar as the bad guy, but long-term high insulin is also a sign of metabolic breakdown. Both scenarios pave the way for neuropathy development. Understanding this underscores the need to treat the root cause, not just manage the symptom.

Source:

1. *https://www.ncbi.nlm.nih.gov/pmc/articles/PMC3303591/*

Insulin Crisis: When Blood Sugar Control Collapses & Nerves Suffer

The body can only sustain the overproduction of insulin for so long. Eventually, the beta cells in the pancreas become exhausted and start to fail. This decline in insulin production, accompanied by persistent insulin resistance, leads to full-blown type 2 diabetes – a major risk factor for debilitating neuropathy.

Beta-Cell Dysfunction: Progression of Neuropathy

- **Faltering Insulin Production**: As beta cells fail, insulin output drops, BUT cells are still resistant to its effects. This means blood sugar skyrockets.
- **Nerves Under Siege**: Nerves are now bombarded with extremely high glucose levels. Damage progresses rapidly, often with a worsening of neuropathy symptoms.
- **Inflammation Explosion**: Uncontrolled blood sugar creates a state of extreme inflammation throughout the body, further exacerbating nerve dysfunction.

Type 2 Diabetes and Nerve Health

- **Unrelenting Damage**: People with uncontrolled diabetes experience accelerated nerve fiber damage due to the toxic metabolic environment.
- **The Complications**: This significantly increases the risk of:
  - Severe neuropathy with pain, numbness, and balance issues

- o Foot ulcers and infections due to poor feeling and circulation
  - o Potential for amputations in the worst case scenarios.
- **Beyond Neuropathy:** Remember, this also raises the risk for cognitive decline, heart disease, kidney problems, joint pain, arthritis, and vision loss – all linked to blood sugar dysregulation.

The journey from insulin fatigue to beta-cell dysfunction is a perilous one for the nerves. While managing type 2 diabetes is vital to slow neuropathy progression, prevention at earlier stages is far more effective in preserving nerve health and quality of life.

Insulin Exhaustion: The Dire Consequences for Your Nerves

By this stage, blood sugar control has gone completely off the rails. The combination of insufficient insulin production and cells utterly unresponsive to its signal creates a devastating environment for your nerves.

Unchecked Blood Sugar: The Silent Nerve Killer

- **Relentless Barrage:** Extremely high blood sugar levels now persist throughout the day and night. Nerves are bathing in poison.

- **Mechanisms of Damage:** The key culprits remain:
  - Oxidative stress: Overwhelmed cellular defenses and increased production of harmful molecules (ROS) directly damage delicate nerve fibers.
  - Chronic inflammation: This worsens exponentially, directly injuring nerves and impairing their ability to heal.
  - Direct glucose toxicity: The nerves are literally poisoned by excess glucose.
- **Rapid Deterioration:** This toxic environment accelerates nerve fiber loss and breakdown of the protective covering around nerves (myelin sheath).

Heightened Risk of Complications & Disability

- **Severe Neuropathy:** This means not just numbness or tingling, but potentially:
  - Burning, stabbing, or deep aching pain
  - Extreme sensitivity to touch
  - Muscle weakness, balance problems, increased falls
- **The Pain Paradox:** As the dis-ease process worsens, pain fibers fail to send signals to the brain and complete numbness can set in. This

makes balance extremely difficult and driving unsafe.

- **Impaired Wound Healing:** Blood vessel damage and decreased sensation make even minor injuries on the feet dangerous, with a high risk of non-healing ulcers and infections.
- **Amputation Threat:** In the worst-case scenario, uncontrolled infections and tissue death in the extremities may necessitate amputation.

Diabetic neuropathy unchecked can have a devastating impact on mobility, independence, and overall quality of life. This underscores the absolute urgency of tight blood sugar control for those with diabetes, BUT, even more importantly, the critical need to prevent insulin dysfunction from ever reaching this stage.

ACTION STEP: Insulin-glucagon balance is essential for maintaining healthy blood sugar levels. When this balance is disrupted, it can lead to many health problems, including neuropathy.

See if your blood sugar levels are higher than the normal range. If it's high, then we must get it under control to have a good chance of reversing neuropathy symptoms.

We will test fasting blood glucose and HbA1c. If you are interested in having your blood glucose level tested, scan the code below.

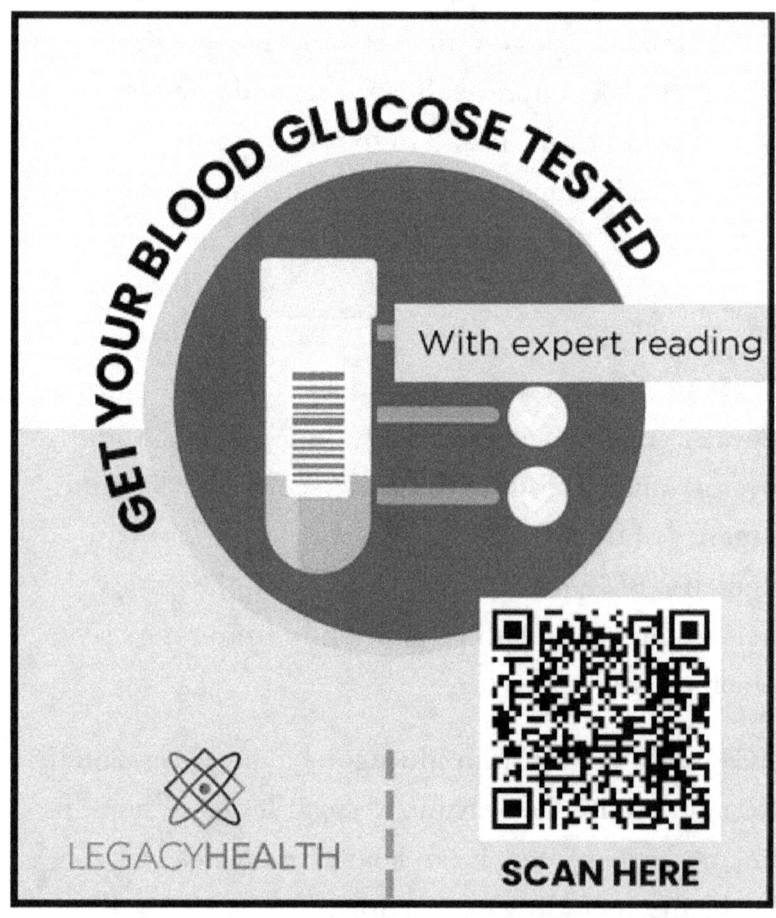

Back on My Bike: How LEGACY Restored Gene's Balance

"When I first started the LEGACY program, my balance was off, and I didn't feel good about my body. I could tell things just weren't the same. I couldn't even ride my bike – I was actually thinking about selling it! People told me to just take something to numb the pain, but I knew that wasn't fixing the problem. It was just masking it, and could lead to even bigger problems down the road.

I decided to treat the problem, not just the symptoms, and that's how I found LEGACY. Following the program and doing the work – taking supplements, exercising, doing the treatments – made a huge difference. I started noticing improvements right away. Now, I can feel different temperatures on my feet, and I've even been riding my bike again!

It wasn't always easy, but the program was definitely worth it! LEGACY helped me restore my confidence and get back to doing the things I love."

** Individual results may vary.*

Unlock Your Path to Neuropathy Relief Now: Call 717-285-0001 to Speak With a Skilled Neuropathy Professional Today!

5

STRATEGIES FOR PREVENTING AND REVERSING INSULIN DYSFUNCTION TO GUARD AGAINST NEUROPATHY

Eating for Resilience: Food as Medicine for Insulin & Nerve Health

Dietary changes aren't just a "nice to have" in blood sugar management and neuropathy prevention – they are the backbone of any effective strategy. Let's focus on the core principles and types of foods that support balanced blood sugar and reduce your reliance on excessive insulin production.

Dietary Interventions for Blood Sugar Stability

- **Eat Organic:** Foods that are conventionally grown are commonly soaked in herbicides and pesticides. These toxins promote inflammation and use up valuable nutrients when cleansed from the body - nutrients nerves need for optimal function. If they are unable to be eliminated, toxins are often stored in fat. Many nerves are encased in a myelin sheath which is largely made of fat. So is your brain. That's not where you want poisons stored. This is why it's so important to eat foods without bug-spray and weed-killer on them. It's worth the investment to buy organic. Invest in your food now or you'll probably have to pay the price with your health later.

- **Non-GMO:** Additionally, Genetically modified organisms are food products whose DNA has been altered from its original design. Because the majority of the immune system resides in the gut, these "frankenfoods" can trigger the immune response to be on high alert; increasing the risk of autoimmune diseases and a host of other health concerns. There's a reason why Europe has banned these foods.
- **Prioritize Whole Foods:** Focus on heirloom vegetables, fruits, legumes, nuts, and seeds. These nutrient-dense foods promote healthy blood sugar response.
- **Emphasize Fiber:** Aim for 30+ grams daily. Fiber slows sugar absorption, preventing spikes. High-fiber sources include beans,

lentils, veggies, berries, and oats- again, get organic. Oats are known to have some of the highest levels of glyphosate - an active ingredient in many weed killers.

- **Protein Power:** Include lean protein (wild game, chicken, beef, fish) several times per week. Protein helps with blood sugar stabilization and enhances satiety (feeling full). When there are budget constraints, this is where to start with organic. Think about it. Farm animals eat lots of plants. If those plants are loaded with weed killers and bug spray, those toxins bioaccumulate in the tissues. You are potentially ingesting a more concentrated amount in the meat.

- **Healthy Fats:** Embrace nuts, avocados, pumpkin, flax and hemp seeds, red palm, coconut, olive and sesame seed oil, and fatty fish. And don't forget about butter. These healthy fats optimize blood sugar control and reduce inflammation. Make sure to avoid these **8 Harmful Seed Oils**- They are linked to heart disease and cancer and create inflammation which is obviously bad for your nerves (and your whole body) .

- Canola oil
- Corn oil

- Cottonseed oil
- Grapeseed oil
- Rice bran oil
- Safflower oil
- Soy oil
- Sunflower oil

- **Avoid Refined Carbs & Sugars:** These are the primary triggers for blood sugar chaos and insulin overload. Eliminate processed foods, sugary drinks, and even white rice and bread. This is essential if you are working toward healing from neuropathy.

Focus on Nerves

- **Anti-Inflammatory Foods:** Prioritize those rich in antioxidants and omega-3 fatty acids, which fight the major drivers of nerve damage. Examples:
  - Berries and colorful vegetables- the more color, the better. Dark blue and purple foods tend to be higher in antioxidants.
  - Fatty fish
  - Nuts & Seeds mentioned above
  - Spices like turmeric and ginger, rosemary and cinnamon reduce inflammation and

lower blood sugar. Garlic, Thyme, Oregano Chrysanthemum, Hyssop Sarsaparilla and Star Anise are antiinflammatory, neuro-protective and also have antimicrobial benefits.

- **Nutrient Powerhouses**: Foods rich in B vitamins, magnesium, and alpha-lipoic acid support nerve health. Include lots of leafy greens, eggs, legumes, broccoli, peas, brussels sprouts.

Your garden and kitchen are your pharmacy! By consistently choosing foods that stabilize blood sugar, lower inflammation, and provide nerve-supportive nutrients, you take a powerful step in preventing or reversing insulin dysfunction and protecting the health of your nerves.

Lifestyle as Medicine: Optimizing Health to Protect Your Nerves

While your diet is foundational, true metabolic health depends on a multifaceted approach. Exercise and stress management aren't optional extras – they have a profound impact on blood sugar control and the underlying processes that drive neuropathy.

The Power of Exercise

- **Enhancing Insulin Sensitivity:** Regular exercise makes your cells more responsive to insulin, meaning less is needed to do the job, reducing the burden on your pancreas. You'll want a good balance of the different types:
  - **Aerobic:** Brisk walking, running, biking, swimming – aim for at least 150 minutes per week of moderate-intensity exercise. That's only 25 minutes per day with a day off each week. True aerobic exercise helps train your body to burn fat for energy and use up the excess glucose stored in your body. To make sure you're in a true aerobic state, calculate your target heart rate with this formula: 180-age= heart rate ceiling. If you maintain your heart rate within 10 beats of the ceiling, your whole sugar handling system will become more efficient and your nerves will thank you.
  - **Resistance Training:** Building muscle mass improves insulin sensitivity even further. Include strength training a few times per week. Do your aerobic warm-up first to avoid injury. Don't be afraid to work with a knowledgeable trainer.

- **More than Blood Sugar:** Exercise also combats inflammation, improves circulation to nerves, improves mitochondrial function critical for burning glucose for energy production and promotes a healthy weight – all key for neuropathy prevention.
- **Professional Applied Kinesiologists** are trained to test for aerobic/ anaerobic imbalances. They can help guide you in what type of exercise to focus on for optimal outcomes.

Stress Less, Protect More

- **The Stress-Blood Sugar Connection:** Chronic stress triggers the release of cortisol, which raises blood sugar and impairs insulin function.
- **Nerve Impact:** Stress hormones themselves can be damaging to nerves, further adding to the problem.
- **Taming the Tension:** Stress management is essential:
  - **Mind-Body Techniques:** Deep breathing, mindfulness, yoga, and the Neuro Emotional Technique are researched to resolve the physiological effects of mind-

body stress. Heart Math is another great tool. Vagus nerve activities are proving very beneficial. Techniques and guides are provided at our in-person workshops.

- **Enjoyable Activities:** Reduce stress hormones through things you love. Equestrian activities are helpful for many. Creative, imaginative and artistic endeavors are shown to promote healing. Laughter is good medicine. Whatever healthy choices that help you get a deep belly laugh is always a good idea.

- **Prioritizing Sleep:** Essential for balancing stress response and blood sugar regulation. Additionally, the brain does a deep cleaning with proper sleep. For ideal sleep hormones, complete darkness is best. Use an eye mask or unplug or cover any lights including digital clocks and gadgets. Avoid screens after dark and consider using blue-blocking glasses while on the computer.

- **Electro magnetic fields:** turn off wifi and keep phones and electronics far away from you while sleeping. This alone can improve your sleep quality.

Lifestyle factors operate synergistically. Combining healthy eating with exercise and stress reduction creates a powerful defense against insulin dysfunction, lowering your risk of neuropathy and optimizing your overall health.

Finding the Root: Functional Medicine for Neuropathy Prevention

While lifestyle changes are essential, for some individuals, further investigation is needed to identify and treat the specific drivers of their insulin dysfunction. A functional medicine approach does just that, providing a tailored roadmap to restore metabolic balance and protect your nerves.

Beyond Standard Testing

- **Comprehensive Evaluation:** Instead of just isolated blood sugar checks, functional medicine looks at:
    - **Advanced Blood Sugar Markers:** Oral glucose tolerance tests, HbA1c (3-month average), and fasting insulin levels offer more insight.
    - **Inflammation Markers:** High-sensitivity CRP and others assess the degree of inflammation contributing to the problem.

- ○ **Micronutrient Testing:** Deficiencies in B vitamins, magnesium, chromium, vanadium, lipoic acid, and others can impair blood sugar control.
- ○ **Gut Health:** Imbalances in gut flora worsen inflammation and blood sugar regulation.
- **Looking for Triggers:** A Professional Applied Kinesiologist can use functional medicine, manual muscle testing and other diagnostics to work with you to identify unique factors contributing to your insulin dysfunction: food intolerances, hidden infections, hormone imbalances, toxins, heavy metals and electromagnetic stress etc.

Personalized Treatment Plans

- **Targeted Nutrition:** Based on your testing, a detailed eating plan is designed, going beyond general healthy eating guidelines.
- **Supplementation When Needed:** Deficiencies are corrected, and additional nutrients may be utilized for blood sugar support and its associated body systems (berberine, chromium, specific B vitamins, Lipoic Acid and Fatty acids etc.).

- **Addressing Root Causes:** Treatment may include gut health protocols, strategies to optimize sleep, hormone balancing, or targeted stress support.
- **Collaborative Approach:** Applied Kinesiology and Functional medicine empower you while providing guidance as you implement changes.

If you suspect your neuropathy risk stems from more complex metabolic issues, Applied Kinesiology with a functional medicine approach offers a comprehensive, personalized path toward identifying the root causes and developing a targeted treatment plan.

It's Personal: Why Individualized Care is Key for Neuropathy Prevention

While broad recommendations for healthy eating, exercise, and stress management offer a solid foundation, the underlying causes of blood sugar dysfunction and neuropathy risk vary between individuals. To be truly effective, prevention strategies need to be adjusted to your unique needs.

Why Differences Matter

- **Metabolic Variations:** Our bodies respond to foods and lifestyle choices in slightly different ways. There are four basic body types determined by glandular dominance: Pituitary, Thyroid, Adrenal and Gonads. Someone might thrive on a lower-carb diet, while another does well with moderate whole grains.

- **Gut Health:** Imbalances in your gut microbiome affect your blood sugar response and inflammation levels, making personalized dietary shifts non-negotiable.
- **Genetics:** Certain genes influence how susceptible you are to insulin resistance and blood sugar fluctuations.
- **Other Root Causes:** From nutrient deficiencies to thyroid imbalances, functional medicine coupled with Applied Kinesiology can uncover drivers of metabolic dysfunction specific to YOU.

The Benefits of Tailored Support

- **Faster Progress:** Addressing your specific imbalances leads to quicker and more sustainable blood sugar improvements, protecting nerve health.
- **Avoid Frustration:** A personalized plan avoids the trial-and-error of generic advice that might not resonate with your unique body.

- **Long-Term Success**: Understanding your individual needs empowers you to make lasting lifestyle changes and truly safeguard your health for years to come.

While broad guidelines are a starting point, optimal nerve health and neuropathy prevention often require a deeper, more personalized approach that addresses the complex interplay of factors contributing to your blood sugar dysregulation and other specific metabolic challenges.

Transformation Stories: How Optimizing Blood Sugar Protects Nerves

Knowledge is important, but sometimes seeing how others succeeded in safeguarding their health sparks the motivation to take action. Let's explore a few examples, highlighting diverse scenarios.

Case Study 1: Prediabetes Reversal

- **The Patient**: A middle-aged individual with early warning signs – elevated fasting blood sugar, belly fat, and family history of diabetes.
- **The Intervention**: Diet overhaul focusing on whole foods, stress reduction techniques including ventral vagus regulation and NET,

and resistance training. Supplements to correct nutrient deficiencies.

- **The Outcome:** Reversed prediabetes markers- normalized A1c, fasting blood sugar and lipid profile ratios, lost weight, improved energy. Significantly reduced their risk of neuropathy.

Case Study 2: Beyond the Numbers

- **The Patient:** Someone with blood sugar in the "normal" range yet experiencing early neuropathy symptoms, fatigue, and cravings.
- **The Intervention:** Advanced blood sugar testing revealed post-meal spikes. Dietary adjustments to balance meals, plus targeted exercise, gut dysbiosis correction and balancing stress physiology with NET, were key.
- **The Outcome:** Stabilized blood sugar reduced neuropathy symptoms, improved energy, and created better overall health.

Case Study 3: Functional Medicine Success

- **The Patient:** A person struggling with constant fatigue, brain fog, and signs of insulin resistance despite healthy habits.

- **The Intervention:** Functional medicine and AK workup found gut dysbiosis from candida and molds, hormonal imbalances, and food sensitivities contributing to metabolic issues.
- **The Outcome:** A comprehensive treatment plan addressed the root causes, leading to both blood sugar optimization and improvement in neuropathy symptoms.

These stories demonstrate that stabilizing blood sugar is within reach, regardless of your starting point. They also illustrate the need for personalized approaches to uncover and address the specific drivers of neuropathy risk.

ACTION STEP: Scan the code below to download our 25 Anti-Inflammatory Recipes Guide.

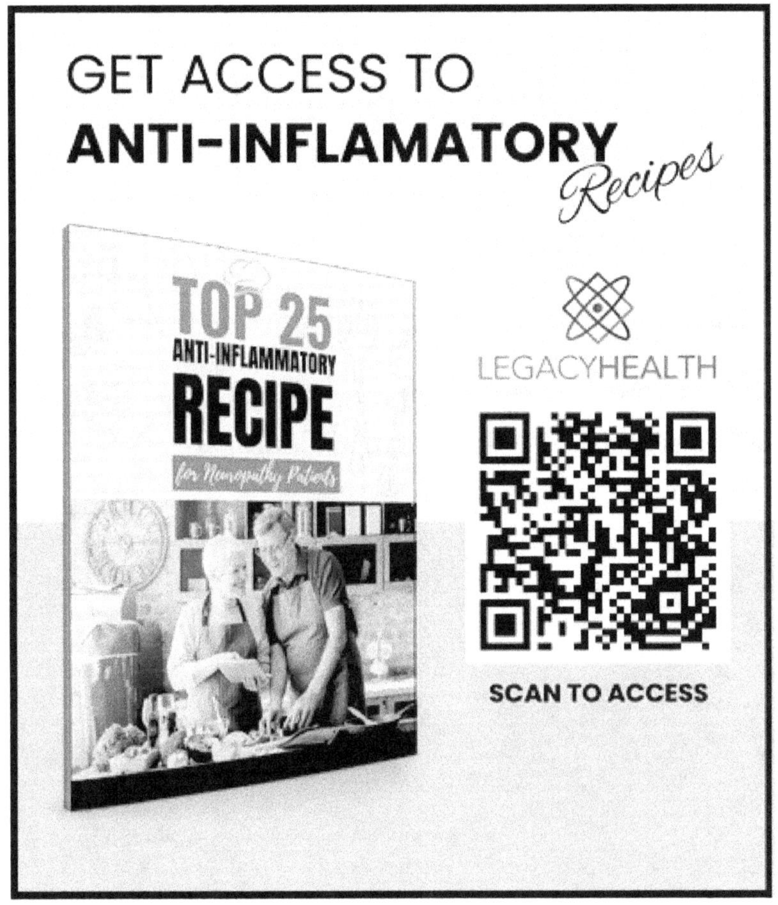

Betty's Restful Nights: Finding Relief from the Icy Grip of Neuropathy

"When I first started the LEGACY program, my neuropathy was causing extreme restlessness at night. The pain in my toes was especially bad, a strange, hard-to-describe ache. It often felt like my feet were freezing, even though they weren't actually cold to the touch.

After just two months in the program, I'm delighted to say I'm no longer experiencing that restlessness or that awful pain! It's a huge change, and I'm so grateful. I've seen how neuropathy has progressed in my older sister, and I was hoping I could avoid the same fate. Thanks to LEGACY and God's help, I'm doing just that!"

Results are not typical. Your experience may vary.

Unlock Your Path to Neuropathy Relief Now: Call 717-285-0001 to Speak With a Skilled Neuropathy Professional Today!

6

YOUR PATH TO HEALING: THE L.E.G.A.C.Y NEUROPATHY PROGRAM

Too often, neuropathy feels like a sentence – a diagnosis that dictates a future of pain, numbness, and increasing disability. It's common to feel hopelessness. But the L.E.G.A.C.Y. Program offers transformative hope. We understand that reversing or managing neuropathy requires a holistic approach, one that empowers YOU to reclaim your health and create the legacy you envision for yourself.

L.E.G.A.C.Y. is more than a catchy acronym; it's our roadmap:

LEGACY

L — isten Intently to Your Story
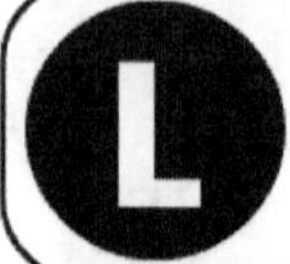

E — xpert Efficient Exam
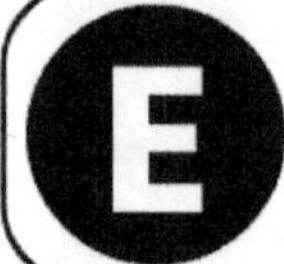

G — entle Genius Protocols
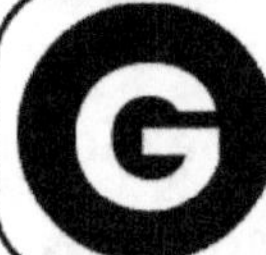

A — ctivate Healing Response
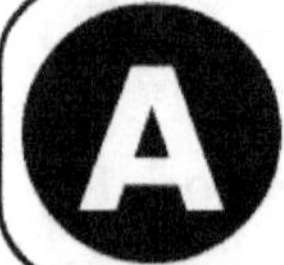
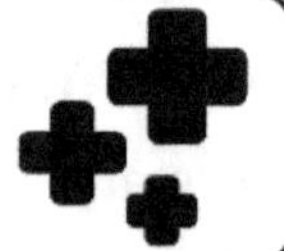

C — reate Mind-Body Connections
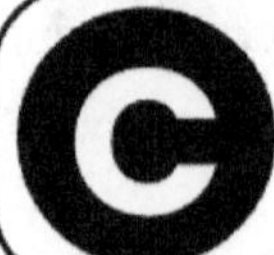

Y — our Legacy Now, You Only Live Once!
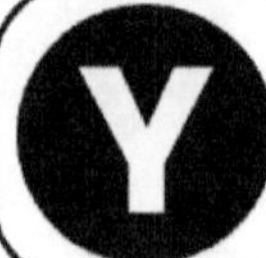
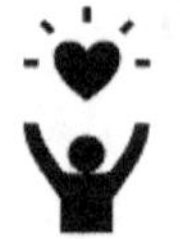

The Nerve-Lifestyle Connection

Your daily habits and choices hold immense power over your nerves. Diet, exercise, stress levels, and more either fuel the processes that lead to neuropathy or create an environment where healing and protection are possible.

For example:

- The food you eat: Sugary, processed foods spike blood sugar and promote inflammation, damaging nerves. Whole, nutritious foods stabilize blood sugar and fight inflammation.
- How you move: Exercise improves circulation to your nerves, reduces inflammation, and boosts blood sugar control. Inactivity increases neuropathy risk.
- Stress overload: Chronic stress hormones disrupt blood sugar, worsen inflammation, and even directly damage nerves.

Benefits of Optimizing Lifestyle

- **Reduced Pain & Improved Nerve Function:** Healthy habits often lessen pain intensity and improve numbness or tingling.

- **Slowed Progression:** Even with existing neuropathy, lifestyle shifts can slow the damage process, protecting your quality of life.
- **Prevention:** For those at risk, these changes are your best defense against ever developing neuropathy.
- **Total-Body Benefits:** What's good for your nerves is good for your heart, brain, and overall health!

Actions to Take NOW

- **Start a food journal:** Track what you eat. A simple plan is to record a section for breakfast, lunch, dinner and a section for snacks and beverages. Do this for two weeks. Notice and record how you feel throughout the day. This can help to uncover patterns.
- **Aim for 10-minute walks:** Small movement breaks make a difference over time. If weather doesn't permit, march in place or try some simple stretches.
- **Basic mindfulness:** Even 5 minutes of deep breathing calms the nervous system. I recommend using the Heart Focus technique developed by the Heart Math Institute to

relieve stress, enhance performance, improve decision-making, and promote health:

- **Heart Lock-In** - perform daily to enhance immune function, lower cortisol, and raise dehydroepiandrosterone (DHEA). DHEA is a hormone produced by the adrenal glands and plays a role in various bodily functions. Notably, DHEA levels decline naturally with age. Some studies suggest that maintaining healthy DHEA levels improves health outcomes, including immune function, stress response, and overall well-being.

1. Shift your attention to the area around your heart.
2. Breathe slowly, mouth closed, through the heart (5 seconds in, and 5 seconds out)
3. Recall a time when you felt love, joy, care, appreciation, or gratitude.
4. Focus your attention on that feeling and feel it in your heart.
5. Hold this state for as long as you can (5-20 mins. is optimal).
6. If your attention shifts, gently bring your focus back to your heart.

- ○ **Freeze Frame** - Use to shift perception and help make decisions when confronted with stress.

7. Recognize a feeling of stress (anxiety, worry, anger, fear, grief, overwhelm, etc).
8. Shift your attention away from this feeling of stress to the area around your heart.
9. Recall a time when you felt love, joy, care, appreciation, or gratitude.
10. Feel this love, joy, care, appreciation, or gratitude in the heart.
11. As you notice a shift in your mental/emotional state, ask from your heart, "What is the most effective/ efficient response to this situation?" or something similar.
12. Listen to the heart-generated reply (perception and insight are broadened in a heart-focused state).

Note: Prayer fits perfectly here in steps 5 and 6. Also, "check your sources" on the heart-generated reply. Not everything you "hear" is 100% accurate 100% of the time or the guaranteed best course of action. Generally, it should line up with the "Golden Rule" and common sense. This is designed to relax the stress system- we all tend to make better decisions when we're less stressed because we have more of our brain involved in the process.

| Heartmath.org, Concepts learned from Dr. Walter Schmidt and Dr. Kerry McCord, https://qahomestudy.com/ |

Remember: Small changes add up to big shifts in your nerve health. Let the LEGACY program be your guide, empowering you to take control of your health journey.

Now let's delve into the first pillar of the L.E.G.A.C.Y. program – the power of truly listening to your unique experience with neuropathy.

Listen Intently to Your Story

Too often, patients feel their story is reduced to a set of symptoms – tingling, numbness, pain. The LEGACY approach begins with a deep dive into YOUR unique experience. This is about more than gathering information; it's about honoring you as a complex individual, with insights vital to uncovering the root of your neuropathy and creating a plan that fits your specific needs.

Beyond the Symptoms

- **Your Neuropathy Journey: We explore the timeline:** When did symptoms start? How have they changed? Previous treatments and their effectiveness? This paints a picture of your neuropathy progression.
- **Lifestyle and Environment:** Daily habits, diet, work, stress levels, and even environmental exposures are potential pieces of the puzzle.
- **Your Goals & Concerns:** It's vital for our team to know what makes it necessary for you to get treatment now. What matters MOST to you? Is it regaining your ability to walk without difficulty? Reducing pain so you can finally get a good night's sleep? Spending quality time with your loved ones? Where do you see yourself in the next 1-3 years and beyond? Your goals shape the treatment plan.
- **Empowerment Starts Here:** Feeling understood reduces anxiety and builds trust, key for navigating the healing process.
- **Clues in Your Story:** Subtle details might reveal an underlying trigger (like a dietary pattern linked to symptom flares or chronic stress that could slow healing) that standard questionnaires miss.

- **Collaboration vs. Dictation:** This isn't a 'one-size-fits-all' protocol. Your active input helps customize the program for maximum benefit.

Benefits of Deep Listening

- **Uncovering Root Causes:** Identifying your unique drivers of neuropathy is essential for a winning treatment.
- **Personalized Solutions:** A plan that truly aligns with your life and needs is sustainable, which translates into real results.
- **Building a Healing Partnership:** When you feel heard, you're more motivated to actively engage in your treatment.

Actions to Reflect On

- **Before your appointment:** Jot down notes on your symptoms, timeline, questions, and what's important for you to achieve.
- **Be open and honest:** Even if something feels minor, share it. The more complete the picture, the better equipped we are to help. We will have some specific questions to help guide the conversation to see if yours is a case we can accept.

Your story holds valuable clues. The LEGACY program begins by turning that story into a blueprint for your healing journey.

Expert Efficient Exams

While your story provides invaluable direction, thorough exams are essential to gain objective insights into the nature and severity of your neuropathy. The L.E.G.A.C.Y. approach is designed for efficiency, ensuring we gather all the essential information to create a personalized treatment plan without unnecessary or redundant testing.

The Thorough Neurological Exam

- Beyond the Basics: A detailed neurological exam goes beyond standard reflexes, assessing:
  - **Sensation:** Testing for sensitivity to touch, temperature, minor pain and vibration, for example, in different areas.
  - **Strength and Balance:** Evaluating muscle strength and gait stability helps pinpoint affected nerves and complicating factors like lumbar disc problems or spinal stenosis
  - **Autonomic Nerves:** When these nerves are out of balance, the body has a hard time

regulating. To ascertain what state the nervous system is in, we may test the 24 cranial nerves for optimal function and 8 muscle inhibition or weakness patterns discovered by Dr. John Bandy, D.C., that correlates to traumas the body is still adapting to. These traumas could include any combination of structural, chemical and emotional factors.

For example, if someone is in a car accident with a front end impact, the muscles in the back will reflexively contract to try to keep you from hitting your head. As a result of the shock of the impact, your stress hormones are released and it's common to experience some fear, anxiety, rage or a host of other emotions. In this example, the body may get "stuck" in extension-leaning away from the dashboard. In the exam, we would possibly see the trunk and neck flexors inhibited.

Resolution of this pattern may involve structural adjustments to muscles, joints and nerve receptors, nutrients to reset the stress hormones and NET for the emotional charge from the accident. Other trauma patterns relate to trunk flexion, side bending, twisting to one side or the other to keep from falling or dodging something coming at us. Diaphragm movement can also be imbalanced because we often hold our breath or tense our midsection when stressed or bracing for impact. It's common to find several patterns simultaneously active because many of us have had multiple stressful events in our life.

- **Nerve Function Tests:** Specialized tests might be employed to assess nerve conduction and pinpoint the type of neuropathy (small vs. large fiber).
  - **Applied Kinesiology:** Manual muscle testing gives us the skillset to assess your nervous system in real time, to determine which interventions are best at this moment and then specifically tailor and adapt therapies and interventions to your body as it heals and treatment continues.

Targeted Additional Testing

- Guided by Your Case: Initial findings and your specific presentation dictate further tests, which might include:
  - **Micro Circulation Analysis:** Through Heart Rate Variability technology, we can screen the health of the micro circulation-

these are the smallest blood vessels that supply the nerves and nerve endings.

- o **Labwork:** Often through blood, urine or hair analysis. We may assess advanced blood sugar markers, inflammation, vitamin/mineral levels, and autoimmune testing if indicated.
- o **Genetic Profile:** This one-time saliva test gives vital information about your particular genetic weaknesses that are often linked to why you develop neuropathy.
- o **Imaging:** While rarely needed, specialized ultrasounds can sometimes visualize nerve compression or entrapment.
- o **Thermal Imaging:** a thermal imaging screening of the extremities is a fast and non-invasive way to determine if adequate blood flow is present.
- o **Consultations:** In complex cases, collaboration with other specialists might be beneficial.

The Benefits of a Streamlined and Effective Approach

- **Precise Diagnosis:** Distinguishing between

different neuropathy types is key for treatment success. But more important is the root cause.

- **Uncover Root Causes:** Did neuropathy arise from diabetes, an autoimmune condition, trauma or toxicity? Or is there some other elusive trigger? Testing reveals answers.

- **Avoid Unnecessary Delays:** Efficient testing means you get accurate information quickly so treatment can begin.

- **Personalized Treatment:** Exam findings help customize the LEGACY program to your specific needs.

Actions to Prepare

- **Symptom Diary:** Keep track of your symptoms, noting where and when they're worse – this aids in the exam.

- **Gather Medical Records:** Previous test results and doctor's notes provide valuable context. As a rule of thumb, imaging and electrodiagnostics within 3 years and labs within 6 months are most helpful.

- **Question List:** Write down any questions you have, ensuring they get answered. A great question to ask your doctor is "What would you do if I was your family member?"

Targeted exams are not about just "checking the boxes." They provide the data we need to see if we can accept your case. If nothing excludes you from care, then exam data helps us build a comprehensive treatment strategy designed uniquely for you.

Gentle Genius Protocols

Generic neuropathy advice often leaves patients frustrated. The LEGACY approach harnesses the best of proven protocols and cutting edge technology that win even where others have failed. We develop a multi-pronged plan that targets the root of your neuropathy and supports your overall well-being.

The Pillars of Healing Protocols

- **Root-Cause Focus:**
  - **Blood Sugar Optimization:** If dysregulation is present, this is foundational, using diet, supervised fasting, supplementation, and medication if needed.
  - **Reducing Inflammation:** Through dietary shifts, anti-inflammatory nutrients, and addressing underlying gut health issues or infections.

- **Targeted Nutrients:** Correcting deficiencies discovered in testing and from our detailed history. These are critical for nerve health.
  - **Structural Care:** Spine, pelvis, feet and other extremities may need to be manually adjusted to correct movement imbalances that impede nerve flow and affect proper gait. Support with home- care devices such as traction or a simple foam roller can help maintain progress and minimize recidivism.
  - **Individualized Treatment:** Addressing thyroid imbalances, autoimmune issues, or other contributors specific to your case.
- Symptom Support:
  - **Natural Pain Relief:** Gentle tapping on specific acupoints on the face can boost neurotransmitter activity in the brain and quickly reduce pain symptoms. Topical creams can manage pain while addressing root causes.
  - **Improved Sleep:** Essential for nerve healing and reducing symptom severity. Sleep hygiene and natural aids are employed.

○ **Therapies:** Based on your type of neuropathy, certain physical therapy modalities to help with balance, for example, or Tissue regenerative technologies may be employed. Additionally, certain therapies may need to be avoided due to surgically implanted devices or other limitations.

Beyond Pills & Procedures

- **Lifestyle is Medicine:** Diet, exercise, and stress management recommendations are tailored, empowering YOU to impact your healing.
- **Mindset Support:** Coping tools and guidance for dealing with the emotional impact of neuropathy are essential.
- **Accountability & Progress:** Regular check-ins ensure modifications along the way, optimizing your journey.

The Benefits of Gentle Genius Protocols

- **Sustainable Results:** By addressing the root cause, improvements are more impactful and lasting than just masking symptoms.

- **Improved Overall Health:** Many interventions benefit your heart health, and energy, and reduce the risk of further complications.
- **Empowered Healing:** You become an active partner, armed with knowledge and tools to support your ongoing well-being.

Actions for Success

- **Openness to Change:** Be willing to explore new foods, supplements, or lifestyle shifts that support your healing.
- **Consistency is Key:** Treatment is a process – steadfast commitment leads to transformative results.
- **Track Progress:** Celebrate small wins to fuel motivation! Symptom tracking and periodic retesting help you see gains.

Your LEGACY protocol is a dynamic roadmap. We combine proven strategies with cutting-edge therapies, always guided by your individual needs and progress.

Activate Healing Response

Your body has a remarkable capacity to heal, but sometimes it needs the right support and conditions.

This element of the program focuses on optimizing the environment for nerve regeneration, utilizing techniques that harness your body's natural healing processes.

Optimizing the Healing Environment

- **Balancing the Nervous System:** Generally, our nervous system has a gas and a brake, the sympathetic and parasympathetic nervous systems respectively. The sympathetic system or "gas" allows us to mobilize energy and hormones to fight, run or freeze. Many lifestyles, diets and the neuropathic pain of those suffering with neuropathy are stuck in a sympathetic drive. This is the survival mode. Your body is not in an optimal state for healing if this system is consistently being taxed and triggered to respond.. On the other hand, the parasympathetic is known as the resting and digesting system. This state is much more conducive for healing and nerve repair. When you feel at ease and relaxed, your body can recover much better. Our gentle genius protocols start with this concept in mind.
- **Blood Sugar Balance:** Regardless of neuropathy causation, stable blood sugar is

foundational and non-negotiable. It's a must for reducing nerve damage and fostering repair.

- **Robust Circulation:** Exercise, therapies, and targeted supplements can enhance blood flow to nourish damaged nerves.
- **Quelling Inflammation:** Chronic inflammation hinders healing. Dietary changes, stress reduction, and specific natural anti-inflammatories play key roles.
- **Cellular Support:** Antioxidants (from foods and supplements) help counteract oxidative stress that hampers nerve regeneration.

Harnessing Regenerative Therapies

- **Beyond Symptom Relief:** Certain therapies directly stimulate nerve repair and restoration of healthy circulation and often reduce pain for many types of neuropathy. Examples include:
  - **Specialized Light Therapy:** Certain wavelengths of light increase blood flow to nerves and promote mitochondrial function for more energy production and regeneration.
  - **Focused Exercise:** Specific types of exercise

can trigger the release of growth factors aiding in nerve health.

- **Pulsed Electromagnetic Field Therapy:** Research shows that PEMF helps improve vascular damage and complications from blood sugar problems, stimulates neurite outgrowth and reduces inflammation. Other benefits include normalizing the electrical gradient on the cell membrane. This keeps cells from haphazardly depolarizing leading to many neuropathy symptoms. Additionally, PEMF helps with nutrient delivery and waste removal from the cells.

- **SoftWave Tissue Regeneration Technology (TRT):** An FDA-approved technology, uses high-energy sound waves which trigger a healing response in the body. SoftWave TRT Decreases Pain, Reduces apoptosis (programmed cell death), Triggers nerve regeneration after injury, Activates stem cells in the treated area, Relieves acute inflammation & modulates the inflammatory response, Angiogenesis (new blood vessel formation), Improves wound healing. Softwave has been shown to increase blood flow by 300%.

- **Digital Electrotherapeutic Stimulation:** Nerves are retrained to fire properly with this technology. It promotes normal healthy sensory and motor function. It is used around the globe and exclusively by the Cancer Treatment Centers of America to treat chemo-induced neuropathy.
- **Other Emerging Therapies:** Regenerative medicine is an evolving field; we'll discuss options best suited to your case.

Benefits of Activating Healing

- **Faster & More Complete Recovery:** Creating optimal healing conditions allows your body to do its best work.
- **Enhanced Treatment Effectiveness:** This maximizes results from other LEGACY components (diet, supplements, etc.).
- **Reduced Pain:** As nerves heal, pain often naturally lessens, improving quality of life. In some cases, especially those experiencing numbness, nerve pain may increase for a time because the C fibers or pain nerves tend to heal first. This can be a miserable phase to work

through, but it is a good sign that treatment is working and it will resolve as the body heals and other nerves come back online.

Actions for Activation

- **Prioritize Healing Foods:** Load up on fruits, vegetables, and anti-inflammatory spices to provide the building blocks for repair.
- **Mindful Movement:** Start with small, achievable actions and gradually increase activity as tolerated.
- **Discuss Regenerative Options:** Ask about specific therapies that might benefit your type of neuropathy.

The Takeaway: Your body is designed to heal! The LEGACY program provides the right combination of support, strategies, and targeted therapies to remove the interference, awaken this potential and promote lasting improvement.

Create Mind-Body Connections

Neuropathy impacts you not just physically, but also mentally and emotionally. Pain, uncertainty, and lifestyle limitations can create a cycle of stress that worsens symptoms and hampers healing. The LEGACY program emphasizes the mind-body connection, providing tools to break this cycle and cultivate resilience.

The Stress-Neuropathy Cycle

- **Stress Worsens Pain:** Stress hormones directly sensitize nerves, making pain more intense.
- **Mental Anguish:** Feeling overwhelmed, worried, or frustrated is common with neuropathy, but this fuels further stress.
- **Impact on Healing:** Chronic stress impairs the body's ability to repair itself, slowing progress.

Mind-Body Tools for Transformation

- **Mindfulness Techniques:** Practices like deep breathing, First Aid Stress Tool or F.A.S.T. (https://firstaidstresstool.com/), meditation, and guided visualization help calm the nervous system.
- **Pain-Management Strategies:** Learning techniques to shift your focus away from pain can significantly reduce its intensity.
- **Emotional Support:** Tools for coping with anxiety, fear, and frustration are essential for

navigating challenges. NET can be transformative here.

- **Reframing Your Mindset**: Working to shift from negativity to a mindset of empowerment and hope.

Benefits of Mind-Body Focus

- **Reduced Pain & Improved Sleep**: Techniques directly decrease pain perception and make sleep more restful.
- **Greater Coping Skills**: You learn to manage stress more effectively, preventing symptom flare-ups.
- **Enhanced Motivation**: Feeling mentally stronger fuels your commitment to necessary lifestyle changes.
- **Boosted Quality of Life**: When the mind is calm, you can focus on what truly matters, despite limitations.

Actions to Connect

- **Start Small**: Even 5 minutes of deep breathing daily makes a difference. Choose a technique that resonates with you.

- **Seek Support:** Counseling or support groups provide emotional support during challenging times. Find a certified NET practitioner here - https://www.netmindbody.com/
- **Celebrate Progress:** Acknowledge the mental shifts you make alongside physical improvements.

Your mind is a powerful ally in the healing process. The LEGACY program helps you harness this power, leading to increased well-being and a better quality of life, regardless of your neuropathy stage.

Your Legacy Now, You Only Live Once!

The LEGACY program isn't just about managing neuropathy; it's about unlocking the potential for a life filled with more vitality, purpose, and joy. This final element focuses on taking those first steps, staying motivated, and celebrating wins along your unique path to healing.

The Urgency of Now

- **No Time to Waste:** Neuropathy tends to progress. The earlier you take action, the greater your control over its trajectory.

- **Prevention Matters:** Even if you don't currently have neuropathy, this knowledge empowers you to protect your health for the long term.
- **You Deserve to Thrive:** Pain, limitations, and anxiety don't have to define your story. Choose to invest in yourself.

Your Transformational Journey

- **Small Steps, Big Impact:** Don't feel overwhelmed by the need for change. Focus on simple, sustainable shifts with guidance.
- **Community of Support:** The LEGACY program offers that support, but also encourages connecting with others who understand.
- **Progress, Not Perfection:** There will be good days and not-so-good days. Celebrate victories, and learn from setbacks.

Benefits of Embracing Your Legacy

- **Reclaiming Your Life:** Reducing pain and increasing function allows you to do the things you love again.

- **Ripple Effects of Wellness:** When your health improves, positivity radiates to every aspect of your being.
- **Inspiring Others:** Your transformation can motivate those around you to prioritize their health as well.

Actions for Today

- **Choose ONE Change:** Start with the diet, lifestyle, or mind-body practice that feels most manageable right now.
- **Find Your "Why":** What motivates you to embrace this path? Envision how a better life feels.
- **Reach Out for Support:** Call us directly to schedule a personalized consultation at Legacy Health 717-285-0001. Please note that scheduling a consultation does not guarantee specific results with the LEGACY program. We'll work with you to assess your individual needs and determine if the program is the right fit for you.
  - Visit our website for more information and to get in touch: getwellandstaywell.com.
  - To learn even more about our LEGACY neuropathy program and reserve your spot

at our next in-person workshop, text "PAIN FREE" to 717-987-7820. This workshop is intended for educational purposes only and individual results with the LEGACY program may vary.

Building a legacy of health is an ongoing process. The LEGACY neuropathy program equips you with the tools, knowledge, and support to create the life you envision – free from the limitations of neuropathy. You only live once. Make it count!

Mike's Back in the Driver's Seat: Freedom from Neuropathy Pain

"When I started the LEGACY program, I was really struggling, especially with my right foot. I had significant numbness, which made driving a challenge – I couldn't even tell how hard I was pressing the brake pedal! At night, I'd wake up with shooting pains in my feet and leg cramps. It was a weird, uncomfortable feeling that just kept getting worse. It got so bad that I started questioning my ability to drive safely.

Now, after a couple of months on the program, those nighttime pains and cramps are completely gone! I'm even able to wear shoes that used to cause me excruciating pain. I'd say my results so far are at least a

7.5 out of 10. It's a huge change from where I was before. I still have some lingering pain, but I feel much more confident and in control of my health. I'm committed to the program and doing my homework, and I'm hopeful that even more improvement is possible."

Individual results may vary.

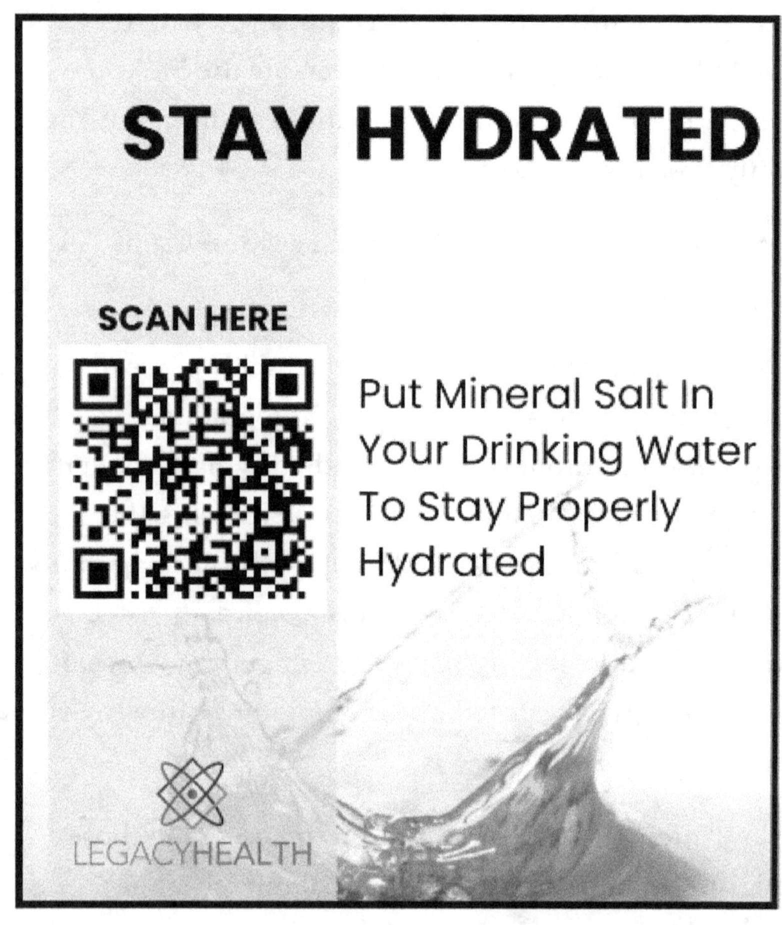

Unlock Your Path to Neuropathy Relief Now: Call 717-285-0001 to Speak With a Skilled Neuropathy Professional Today!

7

APPLIED KINESIOLOGY (AK) - A BEACON OF HOPE FOR NEUROPATHY SUFFERERS

If you're battling neuropathy, you know the frustration of treatments that don't seem to address the root cause of your suffering. You've likely heard promises that fell flat, leaving you wondering if there's any hope for real relief. That's where Applied Kinesiology (AK) comes in - a unique approach that is likely the missing piece in your journey to better health.

Can you imagine a diagnostic method that allows you to test your nervous system in real time and get instant feedback on the results of your treatment? That's exactly what Applied Kinesiology (AK) offers. At its core, AK is about evaluating and correcting nervous system irritation by identifying and addressing "noxious irritants" that disrupt the body's normal function. AK practitioners use muscle testing as a form of real-time feedback to understand how the body's sensory receptors respond to various stimuli. It's kind of like a computer. Your five senses are the "keyboard" and the muscle response is the "monitor" that shows the result of the senses being tested. When an inhibited muscle or "weakness" is identified, it suggests that the body is experiencing an imbalance, and by applying natural therapies, practitioners aim to restore normal neurological function and promote healing.

In essence, AK is a holistic approach that recognizes the body's innate ability to heal itself when the nervous system and its related systems are properly aligned and functioning. Through current neuroscience, we know that the muscle testing response is a direct reflection of the function of the nerve pathways from the body, providing immediate insights into what is needed for optimal health.

This real-time feedback helps fine-tune your care, ensuring that each step is working to restore nerve function, reduce pain, and bring your body back into balance. It's a dynamic, responsive approach that empowers your body to heal and improves your quality of life. That's the essence of AK. It's not some newfangled fad, but a more than 60 year old respected technique with advanced certifications and degrees used by licensed healthcare professionals worldwide, including chiropractors, osteopaths, medical doctors, and dentists.

Dr. George Goodheart, the founder of AK, put it beautifully: "The opportunity to use the body as an instrument of laboratory analysis is unparalleled in modern therapeutics, because the response of the body is unerring." In other words, your body knows what it needs - AK just helps translate that knowledge into a plan for healing.

But AK isn't a one-trick pony. It recognizes that true health involves a harmony of structure, chemistry, and mental well-being. That's why AK treatments may include a tailored mix of joint adjustments, muscle therapies, nutrition guidance, and stress-reduction techniques. It's a holistic approach that addresses neuropathy from multiple angles.

The best part? AK is non-invasive and works alongside standard medical diagnostics. It's not about replacing your current care, but enhancing it. And with oversight from the International College of Applied Kinesiology (ICAK), you can trust that certified AK practitioners adhere to high ethical and educational standards.

If you're tired of feeling like a passive bystander in your own health journey, AK offers a way to actively participate in your healing. It's about tapping into your body's innate ability to recover and thrive. As Dr. Goodheart said, "The body can heal itself in a sure, sensible, practical, reasonable, and observable manner."

For those of you grappling with the daily challenges of neuropathy, Applied Kinesiology represents more than just another treatment option. It's an invitation to rediscover hope, to work in partnership with your body, and to take a step towards reclaiming the life you deserve.

Triad Of Health: A New Perspective on Neuropathy

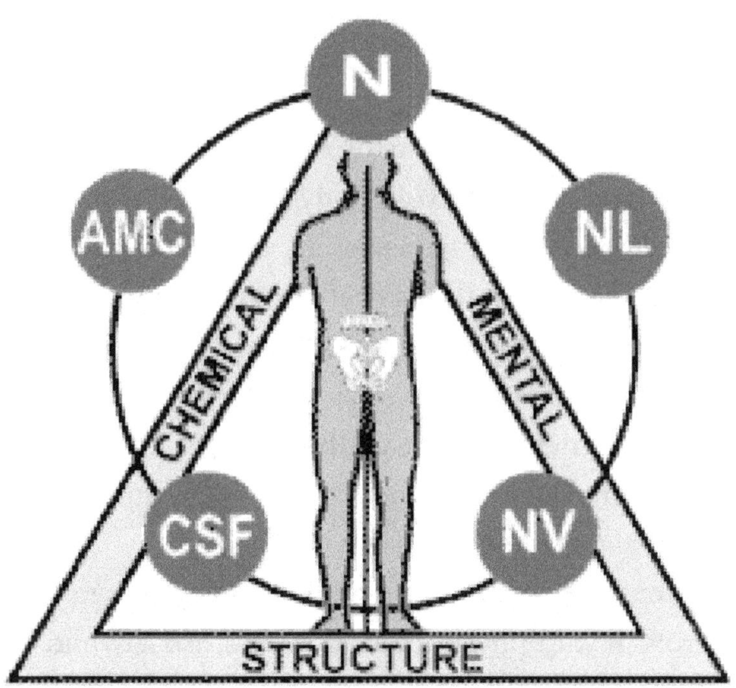

Living with neuropathy can feel like you're trapped in a maze, constantly hitting dead ends in your search for relief. But what if I told you there's a way to see the bigger picture? A way to understand not just your symptoms, but the root causes behind them? This is where the Triad of Health comes in, and it might just be the key to unlocking your path to recovery.

Picture a triangle in your mind. At each point, we have the three fundamental pillars of health: structural, chemical, and mental. These aren't just fancy words - they represent the interconnected systems that keep your body in balance. When one point of the triangle is off, it can throw everything else out of whack.

Let's break it down:

1. **Structural:** This is the foundation of the triangle. It's about your body's physical alignment - your spine, joints, and muscles. Even small imbalances here can have ripple effects throughout your system.
2. **Chemical:** Think of this as your body's internal environment. Are you getting enough of the right nutrients? Are there toxins or chemical imbalances affecting your nerves?
3. **Mental:** Your mind and emotions play a huge role in your physical health. Stress, anxiety, and

negative thought patterns alter your physiology and can amplify neuropathy symptoms.

Now, you might be thinking, "This sounds a lot like what D.D. Palmer, the founder of chiropractic, talked about." You're absolutely right! He recognized that health problems stem from "traumatism, poison, and autosuggestion" - another way of describing our triad.

Here's the exciting part: Applied Kinesiology (AK) gives us a way to assess and address all three sides of this triangle. It's like having a GPS for your health, helping us pinpoint exactly where the imbalances lie. And the best part? It draws from a wealth of knowledge across different healing disciplines - from chiropractic and medicine to acupuncture and psychology.

For those of you battling neuropathy, this means we can dig deeper than ever before. We're not just chasing symptoms; we're unraveling the complex web of factors that contribute to your discomfort. By addressing structural misalignments, chemical imbalances, and mental stressors, we create a personalized roadmap to recovery.

Imagine waking up one day and realizing the tingling, burning, and numbness have faded away. Imagine reclaiming the strength in your hands and the steadiness in your steps. This isn't just wishful thinking - it's the potential that lies within the Triad of Health approach.

What is Muscle Testing?

Applied Kinesiology (AK), muscle testing is not merely a measure of strength but a diagnostic tool that reflects the function of the nervous system. It evaluates how well the anterior horn motor neuron pool—a crucial part of the spinal cord responsible for motor control—activates specific muscles under various stimuli. This technique allows practitioners to identify significant and subtle imbalances or dysfunctions that may not present through conventional medical tests.

Think of it like a finely tuned instrument, where each note contributes to a harmonious melody. In the same way, a healthy muscle should respond optimally to specific positions, forces, and movements. Any deviation from this ideal response can indicate an underlying issue, whether it's a structural misalignment, a neurological glitch, a chemical imbalance, or even a lingering emotional stressor.

AK practitioners like us here at Legacy Health, are meticulously trained to decipher these subtle cues, utilizing precise joint placements, carefully calibrated pressure, and a keen understanding of body mechanics. By challenging the muscle in different ways – testing its ability to hold against resistance, to adapt to changing positions, and to isolate its function from surrounding muscles – we can pinpoint the root causes of the dysfunction.

This diagnostic tool opens a window into the intricate workings of the body, revealing hidden connections between seemingly unrelated symptoms. For example, a weakness in a leg muscle might be linked to a misalignment in the spine or digestive issues. And an ankle weakness could be traced back to a B Vitamin deficiency, for example.

By identifying these hidden patterns, we can develop targeted treatment plans that address the underlying cause of the problem, rather than simply masking the symptoms.

Unlocking Hope: Neuro Emotional Technique for Neuropathy

As a chiropractor who has dedicated a large portion of my career to helping people overcome the debilitating effects of peripheral neuropathy, I've seen firsthand the limitations of conventional treatments. That's why I'm excited to share with you a groundbreaking approach that addresses not just the physical symptoms of neuropathy, but also the emotional factors that can perpetuate your symptoms. It's called Neuro Emotional Technique (NET), and it is most assuredly a missing piece in your journey to healing.

Living with neuropathy is more than just dealing with physical discomfort. It's the constant worry about your future, the frustration of treatments that don't seem to work, and the emotional toll of a condition that others can't see. NET recognizes that these stresses aren't just in your head – they have real, physiological impacts on your body, including your nervous system.

At its core, NET is based on a profound understanding of the mind-body connection. It recognizes that our bodies can hold onto the effects of past traumas and stressors, creating what we call Conditioned Emotional Responses. These responses can manifest as physical symptoms, including the tingling, burning, and numbness characteristic of neuropathy.

Here's where it gets interesting: NET uses a combination of modern neuroscience and ancient healing wisdom to identify and release these stuck patterns. Since the muscle testing response is an involuntary reflex, we can use it to uncover emotional blocks that your conscious mind might not even be aware of. It's like having a window into your body's own innate wisdom.

Let me break down the eight key dynamics of NET and how they relate to neuropathy:

1. **Emotions are Physiologically Based:** We now know that emotions aren't just "in your head." They involve complex interactions of neuropeptides, hormones, and other molecules throughout your entire body. This means that emotional stress can directly impact your nervous system, potentially exacerbating neuropathy symptoms.

2. **Pavlovian Responses:** Just as Pavlov's dogs were conditioned to salivate at the sound of a bell, our bodies can be conditioned to respond to certain triggers with pain or discomfort. NET helps extinguish these conditioned responses, freeing you from cyclical pain patterns.

3. **Emotions/Meridian System Correlations:** Drawing from acupuncture's Five Elements theory, NET recognizes that specific emotions are linked to different energy meridians in the body. For example, fear is associated with the Water element and can impact kidney and bladder function. Additionally, these organs

relate to muscles used in balance and walking. By addressing these mind-body connections, we can promote better overall balance and healing.

4. **Repetition Compulsion:** Unresolved traumas have a way of repeating themselves in our lives. NET helps identify these patterns, allowing you to break free from the cycle of re-traumatization that can keep your nervous system in a state of distress.

5. **The Role of Memory and Physiology:** Ever noticed how just thinking about a stressful event can make your heart race? Our bodies react to memories as if they're happening in real-time. NET uses this principle to access and resolve past traumas that may be contributing to your current neuropathy symptoms.

6. **Manual Muscle Testing:** This isn't about testing strength – it's a way to access your body's neurophysiological responses. The muscle response is never a "yes/no" or "true/false" indicator, and it's never used to predict the future or tell someone what to do. A muscle that tests strong normally may suddenly weaken when we touch on an emotionally charged issue. Your body's responding to a stimulus. In

this case, a physical, verbal or auditory stimulus, showing us where to focus our healing efforts. Although the verbal/auditory stimulus used with the Manual Muscle test can sometimes mistakenly look like a conversation is going on between the practitioner and the patient's body, with NET we are not talking to the body. Instead, we are only evaluating the patient's physiological response to a physical or auditory stimulus. It's like pupils dilating or heart racing under stress. The muscle response is involuntary and automatic.

7. **Semantic Responses**: Words have power. Your body can react physiologically not just to physical stimuli, but also to words and symbols associated with past traumas. NET helps identify these triggers and neutralize their impact on your nervous system.

8. **'Like cures Like'**: By briefly re-experiencing the emotions associated with past traumas within the safe context of an NET session, we can paradoxically help your body release those stuck patterns. Additionally, specific homeopathic remedies developed for NET can support this process, gently encouraging your body's natural healing abilities.

Using NET, practitioners are able to find and correct these unresolved stress patterns with pinpoint accuracy and unprecedented speed.

Now, you might be wondering – can NET really help with something as complex as neuropathy? While not every NET practitioner specializes in neuropathy, the technique's ability to address the stress-nerve connection makes it a powerful tool for quicker healing.

Chronic conditions like neuropathy don't just affect your body; they can wear down your spirit. NET helps address the lingering emotional burdens – the fear, frustration, and hopelessness that often accompany chronic pain and suffering. By releasing these emotional blocks, we free up more of your body's energy reserves for true healing to occur. I've seen on innumerable occasions where symptoms improve after just one session.

Imagine waking up one day and realizing that the constant buzz of pain has quieted. Imagine rediscovering the joy of simple touch without wincing. Imagine facing each day with renewed hope and vitality. This is the potential that NET offers.

I've seen patients who had all but given up hope find relief through this approach. It's not a panacea, but rather a way to tap into your body's innate healing wisdom and address the root causes of your neuropathy – not just mask the symptoms.

If you're intrigued by the possibilities of NET, I encourage you to schedule an appointment by calling us at 717-285-0001 or visiting our website, getwellandstaywell.com/contact. While NET has proven to be a valuable tool for many of our neuropathy patients, individual results may vary.

Also, a wonderful documentary titled " Stressed" digs deeper into NET and its groundbreaking research. It can be viewed on YouTube.

Jay Walks with Ease Again: LEGACY's Life-Changing Impact

Jay arrived at Legacy Health struggling with immense leg pain and barely able to walk. Misdiagnosed foot pain had limited his mobility and joy in life. But the L.E.G.A.C.Y. program provided a breakthrough. Now, his neuropathy is improved, his pain is lessened, and he has regained the ability to walk more comfortably. For Jay, LEGACY was a game-changer, and he wholeheartedly recommends it to anyone experiencing neuropathy symptoms.

** This is one individual's experience and does not guarantee similar results.*

ACTION STEP: Take our free Nerve Damage Evaluation by scanning this code:

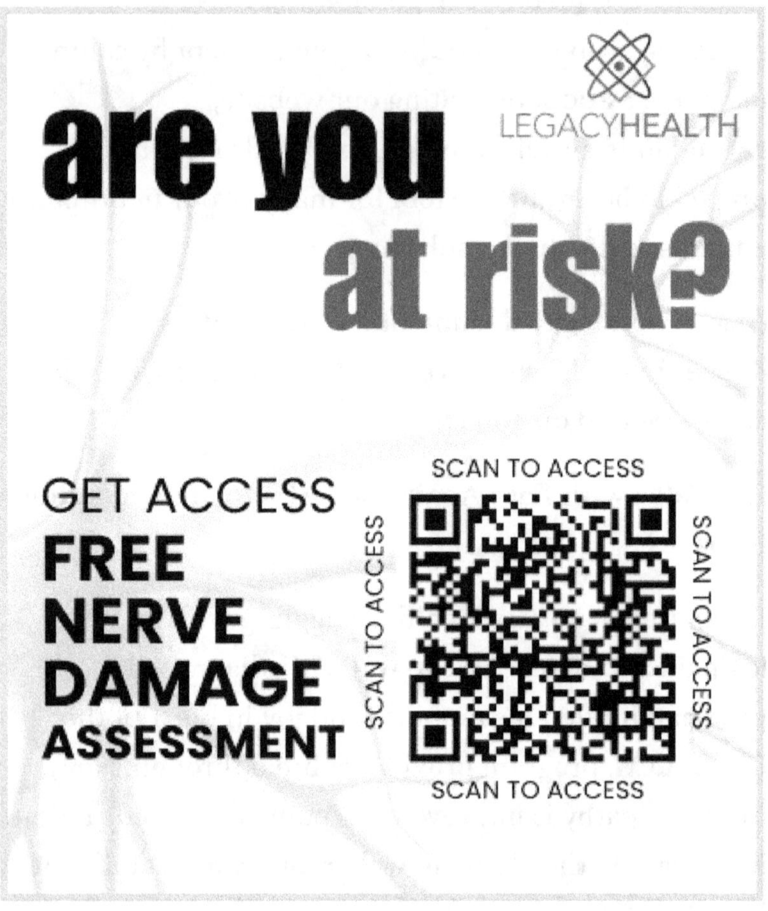

Unlock Your Path to Neuropathy Relief Now: Call 717-285-0001 to Speak With a Skilled Neuropathy Professional Today!

8

THE NERVE NETWORK: UNDERSTANDING YOUR BODY'S COMMUNICATION SYSTEM

Imagine your nervous system as a vast information superhighway, buzzing with signals that control every single function in your body. From the way you walk and talk, to the digestion of your food, and even the beating of your heart – your nerves are the messengers making it all happen.

Unfortunately, neuropathy throws a wrench into this finely-tuned communication network. Think of it like damaged wires causing short circuits. Those signals that should be traveling smoothly get scrambled, leading to the burning, tingling, or numbness you experience in your feet, legs, or hands. But neuropathy's impact doesn't stop there.

This disruption can impact your balance, making walking difficult. It can interfere with your digestion, causing uncomfortable bloating or other issues. Even your sleep can suffer as those nerve signals keep misfiring, making it tough to get the rest you need.

The good news? Your body possesses an incredible capacity to heal itself. That's true for your nervous system as well. While neuropathy can feel overwhelmingly complex, the LEGACY approach focuses on harnessing your body's innate healing potential, fostering an environment where damaged nerves can begin to regenerate and function can be restored.

Decoding the Nervous System

Let's break down your nervous system so you can better understand how neuropathy affects it. It's helpful to think of it in two main parts:

1. **The Central Nervous System (CNS):** This is your body's command center – the brain and spinal cord. They process information, generate thoughts and emotions, and send out instructions to the rest of your body.

2. **The Peripheral Nervous System (PNS):** Imagine your PNS as a massive network of wires branching out from

your spinal cord, connecting your CNS to every organ, muscle, and tissue. It's responsible for things like sensation (touch, temperature), movement, and even some automatic functions like breathing and heart rate. Neuropathy primarily targets this peripheral system.

Now, let's zoom in on an individual nerve. It's like a tiny insulated cable. The core wire that carries the message is called the axon. Surrounding that axon is a protective layer called the myelin sheath – think of it like the rubber insulation around an electrical wire.

When neuropathy strikes, it can damage both the axon and the myelin sheath. With damaged insulation, signals get garbled, leading to pain. Or the "wire" itself is broken, causing numbness. These damaged nerves are why you experience those frustrating neuropathy symptoms.

PERIPHERAL NEUROPATHY

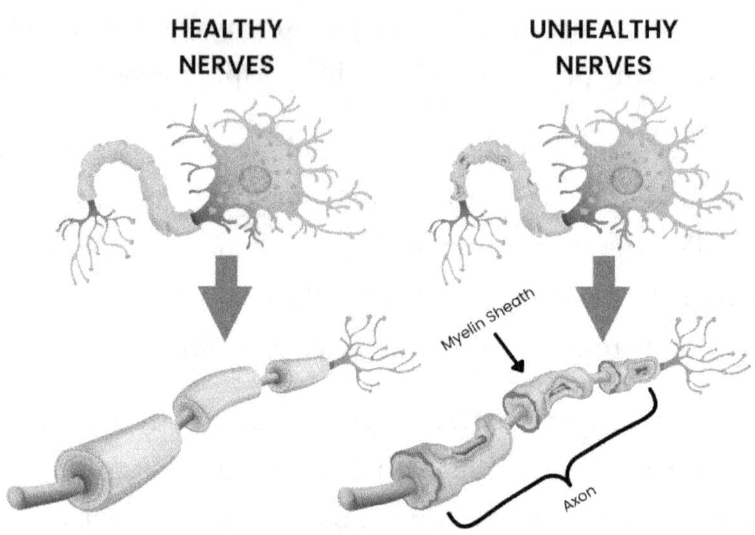

When Things Go Wrong: How Neuropathy Develops

Unfortunately, things can go wrong with those incredible communication networks we call nerves. This brings us to neuropathy, which comes in a few different flavors:

- **Peripheral Neuropathy:** This is our main focus. It's when the nerves in those outer limbs

– your feet, hands, legs, and sometimes arms – become damaged. This is what leads to all those uncomfortable tingling, burning, and numb sensations.

- **Autonomic Neuropathy:** This type affects the nerves controlling automatic functions within our body – things like digestion, heart rate, and blood pressure. While less common, it's important to be aware of.

So, why does neuropathy happen? It's rarely a single culprit. Instead, it's usually a combination of factors that create a domino effect of damage. Let's look at some of the biggest pieces of that puzzle:

- **Unstable Blood Sugar:** Blood sugar spikes and crashes throw your entire body out of whack, including your nerves.
- **Inflammation:** Think of this as a fire raging throughout your body. Nerves are especially vulnerable to this inflammatory damage.
- **Nutritional Deficiencies:** Nerves need specific vitamins and minerals to function correctly and repair themselves. When your diet falls short, so does your nerve health.
- **Other Medical Conditions:** Diabetes is the most well-known risk factor, but neuropathy

goes hand-in-hand with issues like autoimmune disorders, thyroid problems, and even past infections or toxins like chemo.

The key takeaway? To truly conquer neuropathy, we need to go beyond just covering up symptoms. We need to dig deep to identify and address those root causes.

Harnessing the Body's Healing Power

Here's the incredibly good news: Your body isn't a static machine. It has a remarkable ability to heal, and that includes your nerves. This is where a concept called neuroplasticity comes in.

Neuroplasticity means your brain and nerves can change, adapt, and form new connections. Think of it like rewiring a damaged circuit board. While this doesn't happen overnight, it's the foundation of true healing for neuropathy.

So, how do we support this natural healing process? Let's break it down:

- **Specific Nutrients:** Your nerves are hungry for B vitamins, magnesium, and other key nutrients. These act as building blocks for repair and protect against further damage.

- **Lifestyle Adjustments:** Simple things like getting restorative sleep, managing stress, and the right types of movement all reduce inflammation and create a better environment for your nerves to heal.
- **The LEGACY Approach:** Our therapies are designed to directly stimulate nerve regeneration, increase blood flow to damaged areas, and calm that "fire" of inflammation. Combined with targeted nutrition and those lifestyle shifts, this creates a powerful synergy for healing.

It's important to remember that healing takes time and consistency. But by understanding and actively supporting your body's innate healing mechanisms, you unlock the potential for real, lasting improvement in your neuropathy.

Beyond the Physical: The Mind-Body Connection

We often think of healing in purely physical terms, but when it comes to neuropathy, we can't ignore the mind-body connection. Let's dive into why this matters.

Stress – The Hidden Enemy

When you're constantly stressed, your body is in a chronic "fight, flight or freeze" mode. This floods your system with stress hormones, worsens inflammation, and ultimately makes your neuropathy symptoms flare up. Plus, it keeps you in a state where healing simply can't be a priority. You're stuck in survival mode.

Stress Relief: Key to Healing

Finding ways to manage stress isn't just about feeling better in the moment, it's about unlocking your body's ability to heal. Here are some techniques well-suited for those with neuropathy:

- **NET:** As discussed above, NET pinpoints and resolves lingering mind-body stress patterns.
- **Mindfulness Practices:** Simple focusing exercises, like noticing your breath for a few minutes, can pull you into the present and calm a racing mind.
- **Gentle Movement:** Yoga, Tai Chi, or simply mindful walking can be great ways to release tension and improve circulation.
- **Guided Relaxation:** There are many apps or audio recordings offering guided meditations, helping you shift into a more relaxed state.

The key is finding what works for you. Even 5-10 minutes of these practices daily can make a significant difference over time.

The Power of Positive Mindset

You might think a positive mindset is just feel-good fluff, but when it comes to neuropathy, it's much more powerful than that.

The Self-Fulfilling Prophecy

Feelings and actions follow from your thoughts and beliefs. If you believe your neuropathy has you trapped, and that it will only get worse, those thoughts become a roadblock to progress. Here's why. You may feel overwhelmed, anxious or despair. Those feelings can point to an even deeper longing for restoration and wholeness because " This isn't how it's supposed to be!" Commonly shame or resentment can linger for poor lifestyle choices or being a victim to life's circumstances. The actions then, that follow this mindset, lead to giving up, resigning or "what's the point" behaviors that reinforces your original beliefs. However, when you cultivate the belief that healing IS possible, you're more likely to feel buoyant , hopeful, curious, or determined. These feelings lead to healthy activities, resourcefulness and embracing the LEGACY program wholeheartedly.

Mind Over Matter

Feeling heart-felt gratitude won't magically erase your neuropathy overnight. However, it reduces stress (which we know hinders healing), increases motivation, and empowers you to face challenges with greater resilience. It's not so much " mind over matter" as it is that your thoughts generate feelings that actually affect the physical and chemical matter that your body is made of.

Hope Is Fuel

The healing journey can be long. Belief in your body's ability to improve and trust in the LEGACY process can make all the difference in staying committed, even when progress feels slow.

It's important to be honest about the challenges, but don't let fear or past disappointments steal your hope. Empower yourself by focusing on the potential for a better tomorrow.

By now, you have a much deeper understanding of how your amazing nervous system works and the ways that neuropathy disrupts its delicate balance. This knowledge isn't just about knowing the facts; it's about empowerment. The more you understand, the clearer it becomes that you're not just a victim of this condition; you're an active participant in your healing journey.

LEGACY is designed to be a partnership. It honors the complexity of neuropathy by addressing not just the physical damage, but the mental, emotional, and lifestyle factors that so greatly impact your overall nervous system health.

Think of it this way: If your nerves are that intricate communication network, we're providing the tools to repair the wires, boost the signal quality, and even teach your brain and body healthier communication patterns. This multi-pronged approach is what sets LEGACY apart, offering true holistic healing and the best chance of lasting relief from neuropathy.

Kathleen's Simple Joys Reclaimed

For ten years, Kathleen endured the relentless burning of neuropathy in her feet. Simple pleasures like wearing socks or shoes became impossible. She'd almost resigned herself to the pain, but after just two months with the L.E.G.A.C.Y. program, she found herself crying tears of joy.

"I can't even tell you how good I feel! I can put shoes on, wear socks – things I could never do before. My family is amazed at what I've done!"

This newfound freedom has transformed her life. Kathleen's journey demonstrates that even after years of suffering, LEGACY can reignite hope and make the impossible feel possible.

Your results may be different.

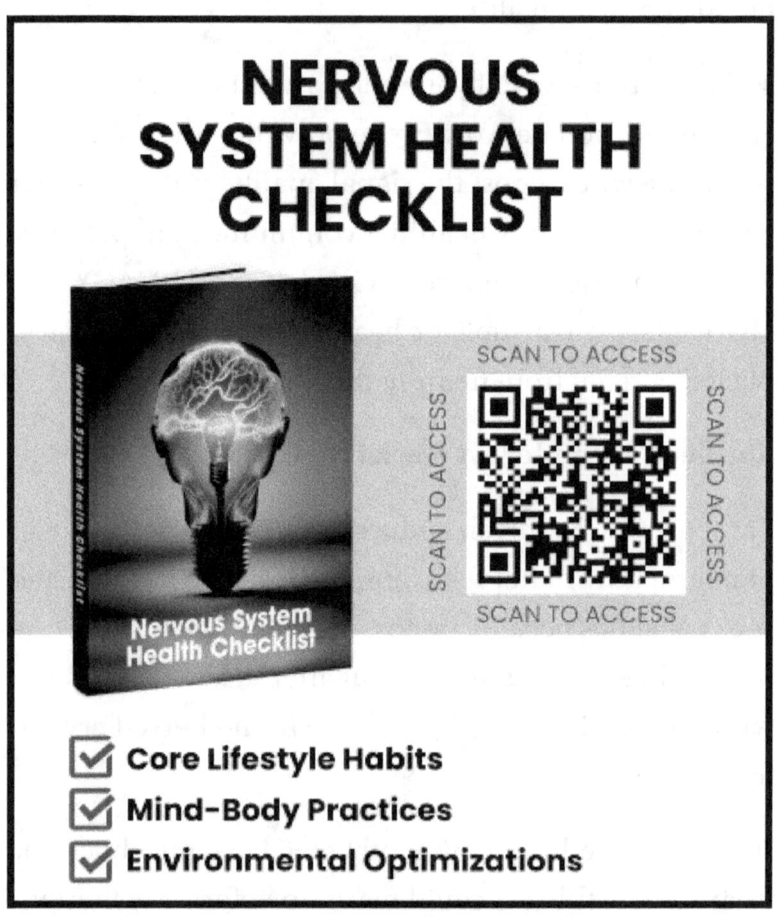

Unlock Your Path to Neuropathy Relief Now: Call 717-285-0001 to Speak With a Skilled Neuropathy Professional Today!

9

THE STATIN DILEMMA: WEIGHING RISKS AND ALTERNATIVES FOR NEUROPATHY

If you, like millions of Americans, have been told you need a statin medication to lower your cholesterol, it's important to understand what that decision truly means. Statins are among the most widely prescribed drugs in the world, making them a critical topic for anyone battling chronic health issues like neuropathy.

For years, the message on cholesterol has been simple: high cholesterol is bad, and lowering it at nearly any cost is good. However, a growing body of research paints a much more complicated picture. It forces us to ask: Are the benefits of statins always worth the potential risks?

This question is especially urgent for those struggling with neuropathy. Studies show a clear link between statin use and an increased risk of developing neuropathy, or worsening of existing symptoms. Unfortunately, many patients (and even some doctors) are unaware of this potential side effect. This chapter aims to give you the knowledge to make informed choices about your health.

How Statins Work (And How They Can Harm)

Let's break down how statins actually work inside your body, and why, despite their intended purpose, they can end up doing more harm than good.

How Statins Lower Cholesterol: Your liver is your body's cholesterol factory. Statins work by essentially slowing down this factory's production line. Seems like a good thing if your numbers are high, right? Well, it's not quite that simple.

The CoQ10 Problem: Your liver doesn't just make cholesterol. It also creates something called CoQ10, which is absolutely crucial for energy production in every single cell. Think of CoQ10 as the fuel for your cellular power plants. Here's the catch: Statins block the same pathway that makes CoQ10, meaning lower cholesterol often comes at the price of depleted CoQ10.

Why CoQ10 Matters for Your Nerves: Your nerves and muscles are incredibly energy-hungry. Depleting their fuel source (CoQ10) can lead to the very kinds of symptoms seen in neuropathy – weakness, pain, fatigue, and more.

Side Effects Beyond Neuropathy: We can't talk about statins without mentioning the broader range of problems reported by those taking them. This includes muscle aches, cognitive fog, blood sugar disruptions, and even increased risk for conditions like Parkinson's and liver damage. While some dismiss these as "mild," they have a massive impact on quality of life – especially when you're already facing a condition like neuropathy.

Statins & Neuropathy: What the Research Says

Unfortunately, research makes it clear – statins and neuropathy are more connected than many patients realize. Let's look at the evidence, and why this demands extra caution in making treatment decisions.

Who's Most at Risk?

Certain factors make statin-induced neuropathy more likely:

- **Existing Neuropathy or Diabetes:** If your nerves are already vulnerable, statins can make them even more susceptible to damage.

- **Older Age:** Our bodies become less efficient at processing medication over time, increasing the chance of side effects.
- **Taking Multiple Medications:** Certain drugs interact with statins, raising the risk of complications.
- **Vitamin D Deficiency:** Low Vitamin D levels may compound the nerve-damaging effects of statins.

The Misdiagnosis Problem

Imagine this scenario: You're taking a statin, and gradually your neuropathy symptoms worsen – more burning in your feet, increased weakness, and it's harder to walk. Most people (and even many doctors) assume this means the disease is simply progressing. This can lead to:

- **Upping the Statin Dose:** The logic is, "If cholesterol is the problem, and it's not coming down enough, we need more medication." Unfortunately, this often intensifies the side effects.
- **Adding Other Medications:** Doctors might prescribe additional drugs focused on nerve pain, not realizing the statin itself could be fueling the fire.

- **Unnecessary Anxiety**: Thinking their condition is spiraling out of control adds mental and emotional burdens on top of the physical ones.

Here's where it gets even trickier: Some patients with statin-induced neuropathy actually DO experience a period of initial improvement on the medication, as their cholesterol numbers fall. This can lull them into a false sense of security, masking the damage the statin is doing longer-term.

The key takeaway? If you're on a statin and ANY change in your neuropathy symptoms occurs – better or worse – it warrants a deeper conversation with your doctor. Don't assume every setback is inevitable disease progression.

Why Open Discussions Matter

The decision to take statins or not is complex. Your doctor needs to weigh your individual heart health risks with the potential for serious side effects like neuropathy. It's a conversation about quality vs. quantity of life, and YOUR input should be central.

Natural Alternatives for Heart Health

Here's the good news: protecting your heart health doesn't have to mean relying solely on medications like statins. Natural approaches provide a powerful, multifaceted way to support your cardiovascular system AND reduce the very things that drive neuropathy progression.

Beyond Cholesterol

Think of inflammation like a fire raging inside your blood vessels. Over time, this causes damage to the delicate lining, making them rough and sticky. This is where cholesterol has its chance to build up, potentially forming those dangerous plaques that can lead to heart attack or stroke. Statins put a temporary band-aid on high cholesterol numbers, but don't extinguish the underlying fire.

Oxidative damage is another key player. Imagine all your cells, including those lining your blood vessels, as constantly producing 'exhaust fumes' from their energy production processes. Antioxidants are like your body's air filtration system, neutralizing those fumes. Excess inflammation and an unhealthy lifestyle can overload the system, essentially 'rusting' your blood vessels from the inside out.

Why does this matter for neuropathy? Your nerves are particularly sensitive to both inflammation and oxidative damage. The same things that put your heart at risk are contributing to the breakdown of your nerves as well. Addressing these root issues isn't just about protecting your heart – it's about safeguarding your entire body, and especially those vulnerable nerves.

Lifestyle as Your Best Medicine

Let's emphasize how powerful lifestyle shifts can be in protecting your heart and nerves. Start with prioritizing an anti-inflammatory diet. This means ditching processed junk and filling your plate with vibrant, whole foods. Think of all those colorful fruits and vegetables as an army of antioxidants, safeguarding your blood vessels and nerves. It's also crucial to choose foods that won't send your blood sugar soaring, as those spikes cause widespread damage – especially to sensitive nerves.

Don't underestimate the power of movement – even if your neuropathy creates limitations. Find what works for you, whether it's short walks, chair-based exercise, or gentle water exercises like water aerobics. Moving your body boosts circulation (so important for those healing nerves) and helps your body combat chronic inflammation.

Lastly, remember that stress relief isn't a luxury, it's a necessity. When you're constantly in "fight, flight or freeze" mode, stress hormones surge, harming both your heart and nerves. Simple mindfulness practices and thought work, deep breathing, feeling gratitude from the heart, schedule with an NET practitioner, use www.firstaidstresstool.com , singing, laughing and playing with others or even taking a few minutes for a relaxing hobby, can make a substantial difference when done consistently.

Supplements: A Targeted Approach

While a healthy diet and lifestyle are foundational, targeted supplements can supercharge your heart and nerve protection. First up are omega-3 fatty acids, found in fish oil. These are superstars when it comes to taming inflammation, benefiting both your blood vessels and those sensitive nerves.

Certain nutrients act like your body's internal blood sugar management team. Magnesium and alpha-lipoic acid are key players, helping to keep blood sugar levels steady and preventing those harmful spikes that contribute to neuropathy.

Lastly, antioxidants are your shield against that internal "rust" we call oxidative damage. Resveratrol (found in grapes, dry red wine and the herb Japanese Knotweed), turmeric (that bright yellow spice), and many others each provide unique protective benefits for your heart and circulatory system. Here is a list I've found to be very clinically useful as they are high in antioxidants and contain neuroprotective properties:

Rosemary, Elderberry, Hawthorn, Ashwagandha, Olive Leaf, Albizia, Mucuna, American Ginseng, Chrysanthemum, Bacopa, Illicium, Golden thread and Dan Shen. Purity and potency matters. I've found consistent results from Supreme Nutrition Products. You can learn more here: https://www.supremenutri tionproducts.com/index.html

Important Note: Supplements are most effective when combined with those healthy lifestyle changes. Before adding any, always talk to your doctor, especially if you take other medications.

Making Informed Decisions

This chapter isn't about scaring you away from statins, but about making sure you have all the information to make the best possible decisions for YOUR health. Let's discuss how to navigate this, whether you're currently on statins or considering starting them.

Don't Go It Alone: If you take statins, stopping abruptly can be dangerous. Cholesterol rebound is a real risk, and it's essential to do so under your doctor's supervision. This may involve a gradual taper or exploring alternatives.

Questions to Spark Conversation

Your next appointment shouldn't be a passive checkup. Here are a few questions to advocate for yourself:

- "What are my specific heart risks, and what are my odds with and without the medication? how much does this statin statistically help lower them?"
- "Have we run bloodwork to check my Lipoprotein Particle Assessment by NMR ?" (Historically, LDL cholesterol, or LDL-C, has been used to estimate LDL levels to assess a patient's LDL-related cardiovascular risk and judge an individual's response to LDL-lowering therapy. Today, a more reliable measure of LDL exists that directly counts the number of LDL particles a patient has using NMR technology.)
- "How familiar and successful are you with lifestyle changes I could make to potentially reduce my need for medication?"

- "If I experience any new muscle pain, weakness, or cognitive changes, should I report them immediately?"
- "Are you familiar with non-statin options for cholesterol and how can we discuss their pros and cons?"

If the answer to any of these is "no", I would be asking:

- "Who else do you know that regularly wins without medications that could advise for a second opinion?"

Sometimes, statins may be necessary. But even then, the LEGACY approach is vital. By addressing inflammation, blood sugar, etc., you're protecting your heart and nerves, and minimizing the potential damage statins can cause over time. It's about smart, integrative care, not one-size-fits-all prescriptions.

Throughout this chapter, we've uncovered how statins work, their potential risks, and alternatives that nourish your entire body. This knowledge isn't meant to instill fear, but to give you power. By understanding your medications, you shift from being a passive recipient of care to an active participant in shaping your health journey.

Remember, the goal isn't simply to lower a number on a lab test. True health encompasses thriving nerves, a strong heart, and a life where medications are a tool, not a life sentence. Balancing heart health and protecting those precious nerves absolutely IS achievable. Often, this means finding the right balance between smart lifestyle changes, targeted supplements, and carefully considered medications when truly necessary.

Rick's Frozen Feet and Sleepless Nights

Rick's neuropathy felt like a never-ending winter in his feet, waking him up five or six times a night with an icy-cold sensation. Even electric blankets provided no relief. The lack of sleep left him exhausted, his life consumed by the constant discomfort. Thanks to the L.E.G.A.C.Y. program, within just a few weeks, Rick was sleeping through the night and his neuropathy improved by 75%. He's finally rediscovering the joy of a good night's rest and a life less defined by pain.

Individual outcomes may differ.

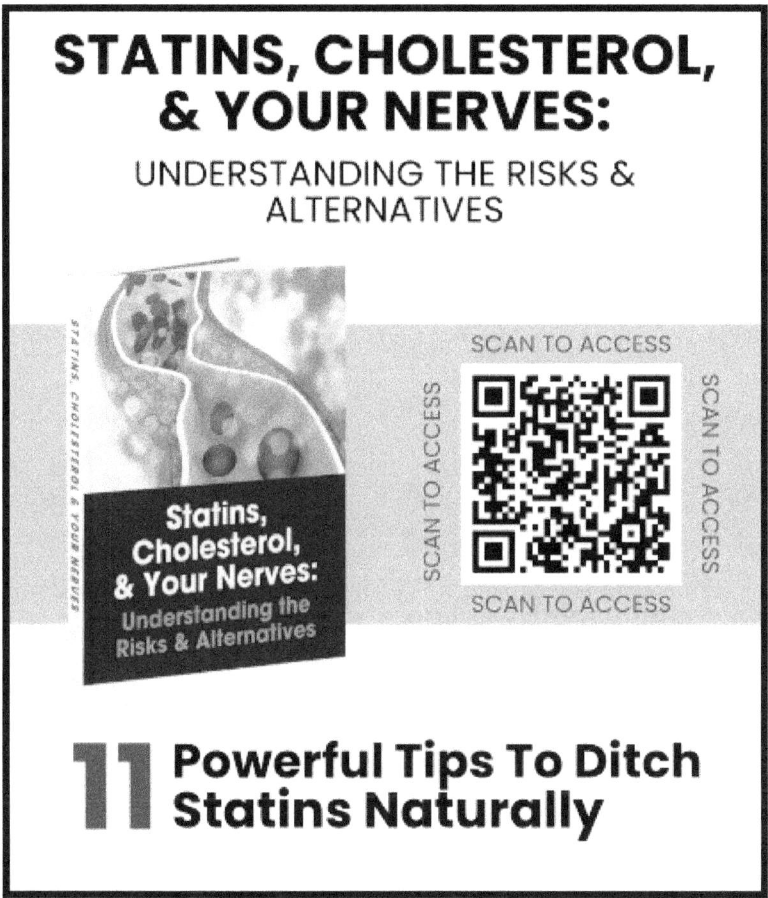

Unlock Your Path to Neuropathy Relief Now: Call 717-285-0001 to Speak With a Skilled Neuropathy Professional Today!

10

ALL ABOUT GLUTEN

The waiting room was abuzz with nervous energy. I could sense the mix of hope and uncertainty in the air – a familiar feeling for anyone who walks through our doors. Many have tried countless treatments, only to be met with fleeting relief or, worse, a dismissive shrug from their doctors. But today was different. Today, I was meeting with Sandra, a patient who had just completed her initial round of the LEGACY program.

As she sat down, her face lit up with a smile that immediately erased any doubt. "Dr. Adam," she exclaimed, "I can't believe the difference! The burning in my feet is almost gone, and I'm sleeping through the night for the first time in years." Her transformation was remarkable. When she'd first arrived, Sandra could barely walk a block without excruciating pain. Now, she was practically skipping down the hallway.

As we delved into her progress, one key factor emerged: gluten. It turned out that Sandra had a gluten sensitivity that had gone undiagnosed for years. Through the LEGACY program, we identified this hidden trigger, and removing gluten from her diet had a profound impact on her neuropathy symptoms.

Disclaimer: Individual results may vary. While many patients experience significant improvement with the LEGACY program, results are not guaranteed. Factors like the severity of neuropathy, individual health history, and commitment to the program all play a role.

Sandra's story is a powerful reminder that seemingly unrelated factors can contribute to nerve damage. It's not always the obvious culprits like diabetes or physical injuries. Sometimes, it's something as seemingly innocuous as a protein found in our everyday food:

Let's talk about gluten – that sneaky protein found in so much of our food. If you struggle with neuropathy, understanding gluten's potential impact on your health could be a game-changer.

Think about how our diets have changed. Gluten isn't just about bread anymore. It's in processed foods, sauces, even some medications. This constant exposure is problematic, especially for those with hidden sensitivities.

The controversy surrounding gluten is real. Some doctors dismiss it as a fad, while others are seeing powerful connections between gluten and a variety of health problems – including neuropathy. The truth is, it may not affect everyone equally, but the research suggesting a link between gluten and nerve damage is too compelling to ignore.

It's crucial to remember, this isn't just about having full-blown celiac disease. Think of gluten sensitivity as existing on a spectrum. Even milder forms can cause significant inflammation throughout your body, and your nerves aren't immune to those effects.

What is Gluten & Why It Can Be a Problem

Okay, let's break down what gluten actually is and why it can become such a problem for some people.

Gluten isn't inherently evil. It's simply a type of protein naturally found in grains like wheat, rye, and barley. The issue lies in how our modern diet has become saturated in gluten, and how our bodies might react to this constant onslaught.

Here's where things get messy: In people with gluten sensitivity, this protein doesn't get digested properly. Imagine it acting like microscopic velcro inside your gut, causing irritation and damage to the delicate intestinal lining. This leads to what's called "leaky gut," where undigested food particles, toxins, and bacteria can escape into your bloodstream.

Why does this matter for your nerves? Leaky gut triggers a massive inflammatory response throughout your entire body. Remember, inflammation is a major culprit in neuropathy.

Molecular Mimicry

Think of your immune system as highly specialized security guards. They're constantly scanning for intruders (viruses, bacteria, etc.), and they have mugshots of "known bad guys." Molecular mimicry is like a villain disguising themselves to look similar, but not identical, to a known threat.

Now, gluten comes along. In people with sensitivity, the immune system notices its resemblance to components of nerve tissue (the mugshots). Coupled with existing high inflammation, this can set off a tragic case of mistaken identity. The immune system, trying to do its job, launches an attack against both the gluten AND the body's own healthy nerve cells.

This double attack worsens inflammation, creating a vicious cycle that can be a major driver of neuropathy for certain individuals. It highlights why managing inflammation is crucial for nerve health, and why identifying triggers like gluten is so important.

Gluten's Impact on Neuropathy

We've talked about how gluten can trigger widespread inflammation. But what does this actually mean for your experience with neuropathy?

Remember, neuropathy boils down to damaged nerves that can't send signals properly. Inflammation throws a major wrench in the works. It irritates nerves directly, making them misfire and causing those painful sensations. Plus, inflammation slows down the body's repair systems, hindering the nerve's ability to heal.

Here are some symptoms that often overlap with gluten sensitivity, making it worth investigating:

- **Digestive Troubles:** Bloating, gas, diarrhea, or constipation. Your gut is often the first place gluten causes problems.
- **Brain Fog:** Difficulty concentrating, fatigue, or mood swings can be linked to gut-related inflammation.

- **Aches and Pains:** Unexplained muscle or joint pain could be a sign of systemic inflammation fueled by gluten.
- **Skin Issues:** Eczema, rashes, and other skin problems are often tied to the gut-inflammation connection.
- **Balance or neurological Problems:** The nerves in your cerebellum are especially sensitive to antibodies that attack gluten. This can cause significant problems with balance and poor coordination of hands, arms, and legs. Additionally, fine motor problems like slurring of speech, difficulty with writing, buttoning a shirt and eating can also be symptoms.

Important Note: Responses are highly individual. For some, going gluten-free brings a dramatic neuropathy improvement. For others, the effect is more subtle, but still a crucial piece of the healing puzzle.

Testing & Beyond

Unfortunately, figuring out if gluten is a problem for you isn't always as simple as a blood test. Let's talk about why, and how to get clearer answers.

The Celiac Limitation

Standard celiac tests primarily look for just a few, very specific types of antibodies. If you test positive, it's a strong indication of celiac disease.

But here's the problem: Let's say those particular antibodies aren't present, but your immune system is still reacting to gluten in other ways. Maybe it involves different antibodies, or a type of inflammatory response that doesn't show up on the standard blood panel. This means you could still be getting hammered by gluten, suffering the consequences, but the test will read as "negative."

The key takeaway? Your body has more nuanced ways of responding than a standard lab test can always detect. This highlights why an elimination diet, where you become your own detective, is often more reliable in identifying gluten as a problem. Keep in mind it can take 3-6 months for the gut lining to heal, and in older individuals, up to two years.

The Gold Standard: Elimination Diet

This means completely removing gluten for at least 3-4 weeks, then systematically reintroducing it. Sounds simple, but there are nuances to ensure accurate results:

- **Total Elimination:** Gluten hides in surprising places – careful label reading is a must.
- **Watch for Improvement:** Track not just neuropathy, but digestion, energy, etc., as many areas may benefit.
- **Mindful Reintroduction:** Pay close attention to how you feel after re-eating gluten. A significant flare of symptoms is your answer.

Other Testing Options: Speeding up the answers

- **Muscle testing:** Through Applied Kinesiology, your practitioner can ascertain the nervous system response to gluten (or other foods). The Muscles associated with your digestion or brain and nerves will typically inhibit (get weaker) when exposed with the irritating food.
- **Taste testing:** One method is to place some gluten-containing food on the tongue and palpate different areas on the body for increased pain and discomfort. If the taste of the food in your mouth creates more pain, it's probably a good idea to avoid it, at least for a while.

Going Gluten-Free: The Challenges

While ditching gluten can be incredibly beneficial, it's important to go into it with eyes wide open. Here's why:

Nutritional Gaps: It's true, whole grains offer valuable nutrients like fiber, iron, and B vitamins. Going gluten-free doesn't mean just swapping to gluten-free versions of cookies and bread. You need to incorporate naturally gluten-free whole foods like quinoa, buckwheat, brown rice, legumes, and a bounty of fruits and vegetables. This ensures you're getting all the nutrients your nerves need to heal.

Social Impact: Eating at restaurants or friends' houses requires a new level of awareness. It's about planning – checking menus beforehand, potentially bringing your own safe options, and not being afraid to speak up and advocate for yourself. Finding a supportive community, whether online or in-person, can make all the difference in navigating this change.

Not a Cure-all: While gluten can be a HUGE trigger for some, it's rarely the whole story. Neuropathy is complex. Optimizing blood sugar, addressing other inflammatory factors, and targeted therapies like those in L.E.G.A.C.Y may still be needed for a full recovery.

Think of going gluten-free as removing a major obstacle to healing. It creates the best possible environment for your body – and the L.E.G.A.C.Y. approach – to work their regenerative magic!

The LEGACY Advantage

Removing gluten, if it's a major trigger, is an incredible step toward reclaiming your health. However, let's talk about why LEGACY is so vital, even after making this significant dietary change.

Healing Takes Time: Even with the source of inflammation gone, past nerve damage may persist. Therapies in the LEGACY system focus on stimulating nerve regeneration, boosting blood flow, and calming any lingering inflammation within the nervous system itself.

Beyond Gluten: While incredibly important, gluten may not be the root of ALL inflammation. LEGACY approach addresses blood sugar imbalances, stress, and nutritional deficiencies, which all can hamper nerve healing.

The Power of Synergy: Think of ditching gluten as clearing the path, and the LEGACY therapies as building a superhighway for optimal nerve communication and repair. Combined, they form a force far more potent than either approach alone.

Understanding how gluten can impact your body is empowering. Regardless of whether it proves to be a major factor for YOU, this knowledge allows you to make truly informed choices about your health.

By addressing gluten sensitivity (if needed) AND utilizing the multifaceted tools of the LEGACY approach, you create the best possible conditions for healing and lasting relief from neuropathy. This combination offers a true path to hope and transformation.

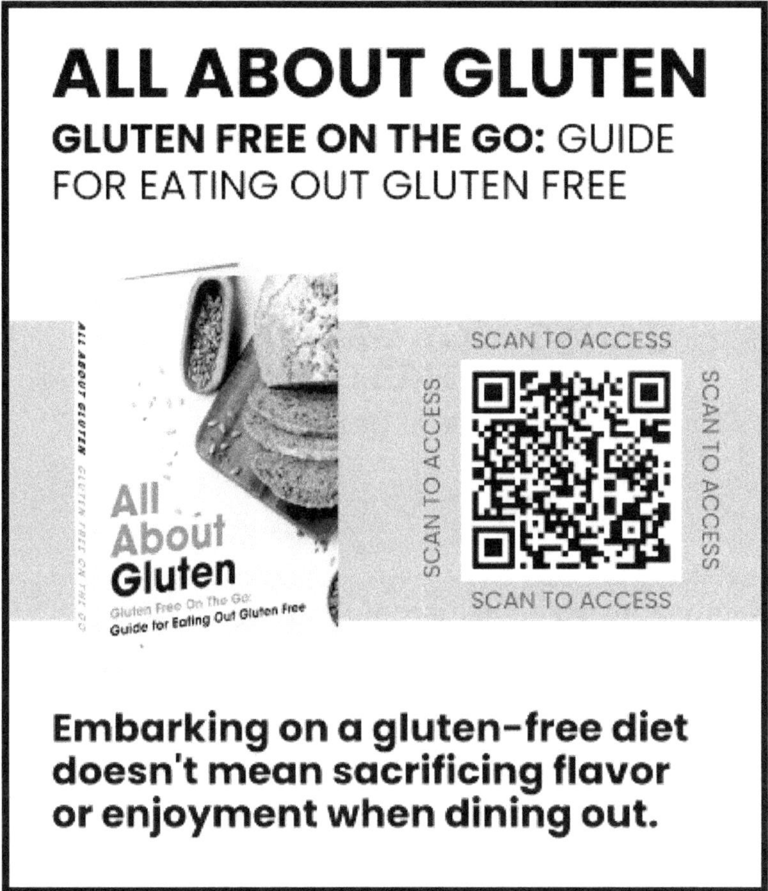

Unlock Your Path to Neuropathy Relief Now: Call 717-285-0001 to Speak With a Skilled Neuropathy Professional Today!

11

———

THE BENEFITS OF HEALING TECHNOLOGY, L-ARGININE, & L-CITRULLINE

Neuropathy is a bit like a complex puzzle. To see the whole picture, you need to address all those interconnected pieces – inflammation, blood sugar imbalances, nutrient deficiencies, and the physical damage to the nerves themselves. This means finding the right combination of therapies and lifestyle changes for your unique needs.

This chapter focuses on several powerful tools that can play a vital role in that healing puzzle: Low Level Light Therapy, Digital Electrotherapeutic Stimulation and other healing technologies, plus the amino acids L-Arginine, and L-Citrulline. While a bit science-y at first glance, these are all ways to work with your body's own natural healing mechanisms. They target those key factors hampering nerve recovery, promoting a healthier environment for regeneration and relief.

Low Level Light Therapy for Neuropathy

Let's shed some light on Low Level Light Therapy (LLLT). Think of it like specialized sunlight for healing deep within your body. LLLT devices use specific wavelengths of red and near-infrared light. Unlike the red glow of a heat lamp, you often won't feel any warmth at all. Other, higher power lasers put off a noticeable amount of warmth.

Here's where it gets interesting: Your cells contain little powerhouses called mitochondria. They're your energy producers. These specific wavelengths of light get absorbed by the mitochondria, essentially giving them an energy boost. Supercharged cells can function better, repair faster, and fight inflammation more effectively.

The science behind Low Level Light Therapy isn't just theoretical. Multiple studies demonstrate its potential benefits specifically for neuropathy:

- Research shows that LLLT can reduce those unpleasant neuropathy sensations (burning, tingling, etc.) while also leading to improved nerve function and balance.

- In lab studies, LLLT promoted nerve regeneration after injury, showing a direct benefit to those damaged tissues.
- For those with neuropathy stemming from diabetes, LLLT demonstrated improved blood flow and wound healing, crucial aspects in managing this complication.

These studies offer compelling evidence that LLLT is more than just a gimmick – it has the potential to make a tangible difference in your experience with neuropathy.

Let's break down the ways Low Level Light Therapy can benefit those struggling with neuropathy:

1. **Taming Inflammation:** Remember, inflammation is a major enemy of nerve healing. LLLT helps calm those inflammatory fires within the tissues, creating a better environment for healing.
2. **Boosting Circulation:** Healthy blood flow is essential for delivering oxygen and nutrients your nerves desperately need to repair. LLLT stimulates new blood vessel formation (called angiogenesis) and improves blood flow to those damaged areas.

3. **Supporting Nerve Regeneration:** Perhaps the most exciting aspect – LLLT appears to encourage the actual regrowth of damaged nerve fibers. It's not an overnight fix, but it offers hope for reversing the underlying damage of neuropathy.

Practical Considerations: How Does It Work?

- **At-Home Devices:** There are various LLLT devices for home use (pads, handhelds, etc.). Quality matters, so look for those used in research studies.
- **In-Office Treatments:** Some practitioners provide enhanced LLLT treatments with greater power and depth of penetration. Complementary wavelengths such as infrared, green, or violet may also be employed to target specific metabolic pathways.
- **Frequency & Duration:** Typically requires several treatments per week, for several weeks or months, to see significant benefits.

Remember, LLLT is like one leg of a chair. It's often most useful and powerful when combined with other LEGACY approaches that address inflammation and support overall nerve health- the other legs of the chair.

Digital Electrotherapeutics: Reconnecting the Pathways of Healing

The nervous system is a miraculous network, carrying signals that keep us functioning, feeling, and moving. Digital electrotherapeutics offers a modern solution for neuropathy by using targeted electrical stimulation to repair, rebuild, and reconnect these vital pathways.

Much like other technology-driven therapies, digital electrotherapeutics works by communicating directly with the body's nervous system. Through precise electrical signals delivered to affected areas, this therapy encourages the nerves to reestablish healthy communication, promoting both relief and recovery.

How It Works: Bridging Nerve Gaps

Digital electrotherapeutics relies on carefully calibrated electrical impulses to "speak the language" of the nervous system. Using a combination of advanced waveforms, the therapy addresses several key areas:

- **Pain Modulation:** By applying symmetrical biphasic waves, this therapy soothes overactive nerves, reducing the pain signals sent to the brain.
- **Circulatory Support:** The inclusion of monophasic waveforms pushes fluids through

the extremities, stimulating blood flow. Improved circulation nourishes the nerves and flushes out metabolic waste.

- **Nerve Communication:** Circumferential stimulation delivers a consistent current that surrounds the treated area, encouraging the nerves to "talk" again. This can lead to significant improvements in sensation, coordination, and function.

A Better Non-Invasive, Drug-Free Alternative

Digital electrotherapeutics offer a better non-invasive, drug-free alternative to address neuropathy and support the body's innate ability to heal. This therapy not only relieves discomfort but also helps the body rebuild healthier nerve pathways. With consistent use, it supports long-term improvements in nerve health while minimizing dependence on medication.

Integrating Digital Electrotherapeutics into Care

As with most holistic approaches, the power of digital electrotherapeutics lies in its cumulative effect. While some patients may notice relief after their first session, the real transformation comes from consistent use over 60 to 90 days. This allows the therapy to progressively rebuild nerve integrity, reduce pain, and restore functionality.

When combined with complementary techniques such as low-level light therapy, the results can be even more profound. Light therapy and digital electrotherapeutics work synergistically to reduce inflammation, enhance circulation, and provide the nervous system with the tools it needs to heal.

Reconnecting You to Your Life

The beauty of digital electrotherapeutics lies in its simplicity and accessibility. Patients can often use portable, rechargeable devices in the comfort of their homes, tailoring the therapy to meet their unique needs. Whether it's soothing pain, restoring sensation, or reconnecting vital pathways, this innovative therapy empowers individuals to reclaim their lives.

Much like other techniques that engage the body's natural healing systems, digital electrotherapeutics remind us that recovery is often about helping the body do what it does best: heal itself.

In-Office Complementary Therapies to Support Nerve Health

In addition to Low Level Light Therapy and digital electrotherapeutics, a variety of other in-office innovative therapies can be integrated into a holistic treatment plan to further enhance nerve health and overall wellness. Each therapy offers unique benefits, addressing different aspects of healing and recovery. By combining these modalities, patients can experience a more comprehensive approach to improving their nerve function and reducing pain.

SoftWave Therapy is a groundbreaking technology that uses acoustic waves to stimulate cellular repair and regeneration. This non-invasive treatment encourages the release of growth factors and improves blood flow to damaged tissues, making it an excellent complement to therapies aimed at nerve repair. Patients often report reduced pain and inflammation, as well as accelerated healing following sessions.

Whole Body Vibration Therapy is another powerful tool in promoting nerve health. By delivering gentle vibrations throughout the body, this therapy enhances circulation, stimulates muscle contractions, and activates the nervous system. It can be particularly beneficial for improving balance, mobility, and strength in patients with neuropathy or other nerve-related conditions.

For patients needing to reduce toxic burdens and promote healing, **Detox Foot Baths** provide a soothing yet effective option. These baths help draw out toxins and heavy metals while improving circulation and reducing inflammation. The warm, mineral-rich water creates a calming experience that pairs well with other restorative treatments.

Finally, **Lumbar Traction Therapy** offers targeted relief for individuals experiencing nerve compression or lower back pain. By gently stretching the spine, this therapy reduces pressure on the nerves, improves spinal alignment, and promotes healing of the intervertebral discs and surrounding tissues. When used alongside other nerve-focused treatments, lumbar traction can significantly enhance overall outcomes.

These therapies create a combined synergistic effect, addressing the root causes of nerve dysfunction while promoting whole-body healing. By tailoring a treatment plan that incorporates these modalities, patients can achieve long-lasting relief and truly get their life back.

L-Arginine: The Nitric Oxide Booster

Let's talk about L-Arginine, a little amino acid that plays a big role in nerve health. Think of it as your body's internal construction crew, focused on building blood vessel highways.

What is L-Arginine? It's an amino acid, one of the building blocks of protein. Your body produces some naturally, and you get it from foods like meat, nuts, and dairy products. Here's why it matters: L-Arginine is crucial for the production of nitric oxide.

Nitric oxide acts like a traffic controller for your blood vessels. When levels are good, it sends signals to those vessels telling them to relax and open wider. This is more than just about blood pressure – it transforms those tiny blood vessels, especially the ones reaching out to your toes, from a narrow, congested side street into a multi-lane superhighway.

Now picture your nerves, especially those delicate fibers in your feet, as a remote construction site in desperate need of supplies. With poor circulation, oxygen and vital nutrients can barely trickle in, making repair work painfully slow. Good blood flow, boosted by nitric oxide, floods the area with everything needed for healing and rebuilding. It truly is a lifeline for those damaged nerves.

Benefits Beyond Blood Flow

Nitric oxide's benefits for neuropathy extend far beyond just clearing traffic within those blood vessel highways. Remember, neuropathy's double-whammy is both nerve damage and the inflammation that hinders its repair. Nitric oxide tackles both:

Taming the Inflammatory Fire: Chronic inflammation is like having constant roadblocks around those damaged nerves. Nitric oxide helps calm this inflammatory response, creating a more healing-friendly environment.

The Regeneration Spark: While research is ongoing, early studies suggest that nitric oxide might directly stimulate the process of nerve regrowth. It's like not only delivering supplies to that remote construction site (your nerves), but also providing the blueprints for how to rebuild.

Dosage & Considerations

While you do get L-Arginine from a healthy diet, when neuropathy is in the picture, extra support is often needed. Here's what you need to keep in mind:

Food vs. Supplementation: While L-Arginine rich foods like meat, poultry, fish, and nuts are great, their impact on your nitric oxide levels might not be enough for significant nerve healing. Supplementation, under the right guidance, gives a targeted dose.

Dosage Matters: There's no one-size-fits-all L-Arginine dosage for neuropathy. The right amount for you will depend on factors like your overall health, genetics and current medications.

Safety First: L-Arginine is generally safe, but it's vital to talk to your doctor before starting. This is especially true if you take blood pressure medications, as L-Arginine can lower blood pressure further. Also, it can alter electrolytes critical for those with kidney diseases. Your doctor can ensure it's the right fit and monitor dosage for optimal benefit and safety. Also, a small percentage of the population lacks the genetic function to properly process arginine. In these individuals, arginine can cause other symptoms like gout, digestive issues and airway inflammation. Also, arginine can promote viral replication. This means it can be contraindicated for those with chronic cold sores, genetal herpes, Epstein Barr or other chronic viral infections.

L-Citrulline: Arginine's Powerhouse Partner

Think of L-Citrulline as L-Arginine's slightly overachieving cousin. It's another amino acid you get in small amounts through foods like watermelon, but its real benefit comes from supplementation for neuropathy.

Why L-Citrulline? Once in your body, it gets converted into L-Arginine - so, it indirectly boosts your nitric oxide production just like we discussed earlier. But here's the surprising part: it may be even more effective at doing so than taking L-Arginine directly!

The Bioavailability Factor

Think of your digestive system as a slightly overzealous security guard. When you swallow an L-Arginine supplement, much of it gets caught and broken down before ever reaching its intended destination – your bloodstream. This means a portion of those good intentions are wasted.

Now enter L-Citrulline. It breezes past those gut security guards more easily, getting better absorbed into your bloodstream. Once there, your body efficiently transforms it into that precious L-Arginine. Essentially, L-Citrulline is like a sneakier way to increase your L-Arginine levels, maximizing the amount that actually makes it to your tissues where it can promote healing.

L-Citrulline's Benefits

Since L-Citrulline essentially powers up your body's L-Arginine production, its benefits for battling neuropathy closely mirror those we discussed earlier:

Blood Flow Boost: That increase in nitric oxide signals your blood vessels to relax and widen. Picture those clogged side streets leading to your damaged nerves transforming into bustling highways. This means improved oxygen and essential nutrients can finally surge where they're desperately needed.

Reduced Pain: L-Citrulline plays a two-pronged role in easing neuropathy discomfort. Better blood flow helps ease those burning or tingling sensations. Plus, like L-Arginine, it tackles the chronic inflammation that often amplifies nerve pain.

Regeneration Potential: Research suggests L-Citrulline might go beyond just boosting circulation. There's early evidence it assists in the nerve regeneration process itself. Imagine it not just delivering new building materials, but also helping create a more efficient construction crew.

Dosage & Safety: Again, dosages will vary based on individual needs. Let's discuss what's right for you, and to rule out any interactions with other medications you might be taking.

The LEGACY Advantage: Synergy & Safety

LEGACY is about harnessing the power of synergy – finding tools that amplify each other's effects. This is where combining Low Level Light Therapy, L-Arginine, and L-Citrulline truly shines.

Think of each as tackling neuropathy from a slightly different angle:

- **Low Level Light Therapy:** Promotes healing at the cellular level, reducing inflammation and encouraging nerve regeneration.
- **L-Arginine & L-Citrulline:** Optimize blood flow, ensuring the oxygen and nutrients for repair get where they need to go.

The result? Instead of isolated benefits, they work together to create the ideal environment for your nerves to heal. It's more than the sum of its parts.

The Natural Advantage

Compared to many traditional neuropathy treatments that focus on masking symptoms or carry significant side effect risks, these approaches work with your body's own healing systems. This means they're generally safe and offer a gentler path to finding relief.

Important Note: While natural, discussing these therapies with your doctor, chiropractor, or another qualified professional is vital. They can offer personalized dosing guidance and rule out any medication interactions. Remember, at Legacy Health, we're committed to an integrative, individualized approach to conquering neuropathy.

We've covered a lot about how Low Level Light Therapy, L-Arginine, and L-Citrulline can aid in your fight against neuropathy. Here's the key takeaway: these are powerful tools that work with your body's own natural capacity to heal. They reduce inflammation, improve blood flow, and may even directly support the regeneration of damaged nerves.

While none of these are overnight miracles, they empower you to take charge of your health. Instead of just masking symptoms, you're addressing some of the root causes that hinder healing. These therapies provide the optimal environment for your body to do what it knows how to do best – repair and rebuild. That's true freedom from the grip of neuropathy.

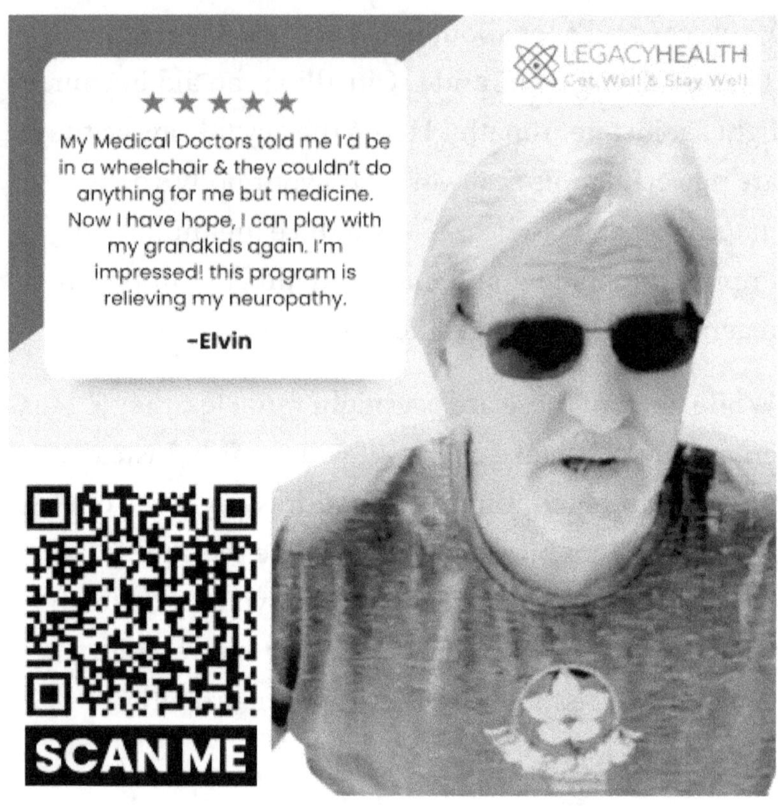

Unlock Your Path to Neuropathy Relief Now: Call 717-285-0001 to Speak With a Skilled Neuropathy Professional Today!

12

A TRUE EPIDEMIC - OPIOIDS

I remember the first time I met Thomas. He shuffled into my office, his face etched with pain, his shoulders slumped with the weight of years spent battling debilitating neuropathy. He'd tried everything: countless medications, injections, even surgery. Nothing offered lasting relief, and he was starting to lose hope.

His doctor had prescribed opioids for the pain, and while they initially provided some relief, Thomas quickly found himself needing higher and higher doses to achieve the same effect. He was trapped in a vicious cycle, desperate for any escape from the relentless burning in his feet.

That's where LEGACY came in. Together, we worked to address the root causes of his neuropathy – a combination of blood sugar imbalances and nutritional deficiencies. We incorporated targeted therapies to promote nerve healing and calm the inflammation that was fueling his pain. And most importantly, we worked on strategies to help Thomas manage his pain without relying solely on opioids.

Within weeks, he started feeling a difference. The burning sensation lessened, his sleep improved, and he was able to reduce his reliance on pain medication. Thomas's story is a testament to the power of a multi-faceted approach to neuropathy that goes beyond just masking the symptoms. It's about finding sustainable solutions that address the underlying causes and empower individuals to reclaim their lives.

Disclaimer: Individual results may vary. While many patients experience significant improvement with the LEGACY program, results are not guaranteed. Factors like the severity of neuropathy, individual health history, and commitment to the program all play a role.

Thomas's experience, though ultimately a success story, highlights a painful truth: the very medications often prescribed for neuropathy pain can create a whole new set of challenges.

We can't talk about conquering neuropathy without addressing the other epidemic devastating millions: opioid addiction. It's important to understand that this isn't about demonizing those who end up in its grip, but about highlighting how easily it can happen, especially with the intense pain neuropathy causes.

The numbers paint a bleak picture. According to the Centers for Disease Control and Prevention (CDC), more than 1 million people have died since 1999 from a drug overdose, and more than 75% of drug overdose deaths involved opioids. It's a vicious cycle – a person in agony turns to medication seeking relief, unaware of just how risky that path can be.

Neuropathy creates a perfect storm for vulnerability. The relentless burning, tingling, or the feeling of electric shocks jolting through your body can drive even the strongest among us to a breaking point. In that moment of desperation, powerful painkillers can seem like the only solution.

While there may be rare situations where very short-term opioid use is necessary under strict medical guidance, it's crucial to go into this with eyes wide open about the risks involved. What might feel like a lifesaver at first can all too quickly become a dangerous trap.

How Opioids Work (And Why They Don't)

Here's the problem with opioids when it comes to neuropathy: they provide an illusion of relief, but don't actually heal anything. Understanding this is crucial.

Think about it this way: Opioids work by essentially blocking pain signals from reaching your brain. It's like cutting the wires to a fire alarm – the fire is still raging, but you no longer hear the warning siren. This provides the feeling of relief, but the underlying damage that is the source of those neuropathy symptoms continues unchecked.

The Tolerance Trap: Your body is incredibly adaptable. Over time, it builds a tolerance to opioids. You stop getting the same degree of pain relief from the original dose. This leads to a dangerous cycle – the person craves that numbing effect, escalating the dose time and time again. It becomes less about managing pain, and more about simply avoiding withdrawal symptoms.

The Hidden Costs of Opioids

Opioids carry a heavy price tag that extends far beyond the risk of addiction. Even when taken "as prescribed," side effects can become debilitating for those with neuropathy.

Physical Consequences

Constipation: Severe constipation isn't just uncomfortable, it has cascading effects. Straining on the toilet can worsen existing health issues like hemorrhoids or hernias. Plus, the toxins that build up in your system when your gut is sluggish can worsen inflammation, a major roadblock to neuropathy healing.

Brain Fog: Opioids cause a fuzzy, disoriented feeling that's more than just an annoyance. When you're already dealing with the cognitive impacts neuropathy can have, this added mental cloud makes it incredibly difficult to work, manage everyday tasks, and engage with the people you love.

Hormone Havoc: Opioids throw off your delicate hormone balance. This can manifest in a whole host of ways – sleep disruptions that make neuropathy pain harder to cope with, low mood and irritability, and even metabolic changes that affect your weight and overall energy levels. It chips away at your sense of well-being, making the battle against neuropathy even more challenging.

Worsening Neuropathy Risk

This emerging link between opioids and long-term nerve damage is incredibly alarming and highlights why seeking alternatives for neuropathy pain is so vital. Here's what you need to keep in mind.

How Opioid-Induced Damage Might Occur: While research is ongoing, several theories exist:

- Opioids may increase inflammation and oxidative stress, further harming already delicate nerves.
- They might directly damage sensory receptors within the nerves themselves.
- By suppressing natural pain signaling, they might delay you from seeking other interventions that could actually help heal the neuropathy.

A Vicious Cycle

Here's why the opioid trap is so insidious, especially for neuropathy patients. Let's walk through a potential scenario:

1. Desperate for relief, you begin taking opioids. Initially, they seem to work, masking the pain.
2. Over time, your body develops tolerance, and those painful neuropathy symptoms start to creep back in.

3. Thinking more = better, the dose gradually increases (often with or without doctor awareness). This offers temporary relief, but continues to worsen that underlying neuropathy long-term.
4. Repeat. More pain now requires an even higher dose, further escalating the cycle.

Because opioids work by cutting off the brain's perception of pain, it feels like they're "solving" the problem. But the damage continues, making you think you need the medication even more desperately. The drug slowly changes from being a way to manage pain, to being the primary driver of your pain.

Breaking free from this cycle is incredibly challenging, as the body has become physically dependent upon the opioids. That's why it's so crucial to address neuropathy pain at its root and explore safer alternatives before the addiction risk escalates.

Breaking Free from The Opioid Trap

While escaping the grip of opioid dependency is incredibly difficult, it IS absolutely possible. It's important to communicate this message of hope, alongside the practical steps and support necessary for success.

There is no shame in becoming addicted to opioids. This can happen to anyone when faced with relentless pain. Recognizing you need help is a powerful first step, and there are resources available.

Safe Tapering is Non-Negotiable

Quitting opioids cold-turkey is incredibly dangerous, leading to severe withdrawal symptoms, which can include:

- Severe muscle aches and flu-like symptoms
- Intense anxiety, restlessness, and insomnia
- Digestive issues (nausea, diarrhea, vomiting)
- Changes in blood pressure and heart rate

The severity of these varies, but the experience is undeniably awful. This is why attempting to quit without medical guidance is so risky. It often leads to relapse simply to ease the suffering, even when the person desperately wants to break free.

An addiction medicine specialist can design a slow, customized tapering schedule based on your individual dose and usage history. This minimizes the withdrawal symptoms, making them much more manageable. While still difficult, the process becomes more tolerable, increasing the chances of success.

The key to lasting freedom from opioids is addressing the root cause of the pain driving their use – the neuropathy itself. Instead of just numbing symptoms, the L.E.G.A.C.Y. approach aims to heal those damaged nerves. As pain naturally lessens and function improves, reliance on medication decreases organically. This offers a sustainable path forward, not just a temporary fix.

Preventing the Cycle from Starting

Let's shift our focus to how we can prevent this devastating cycle from ever even beginning. The key lies in addressing neuropathy proactively and fostering open communication with your healthcare team.

The longer neuropathy pain goes unaddressed, the greater the risk of turning to opioids out of desperation. Seeking LEGACY-type care as soon as possible is vital. When pain is better managed from the outset, the temptation of risky quick fixes decreases.

It's crucial to be upfront with your doctor about the severity of your neuropathy pain, even if you fear being judged. Don't minimize your suffering! This allows us to explore safer alternatives early on – things like targeted therapies, specific types of exercise, or non-opioid pain management strategies.

Battling opioid addiction takes courage, and the journey isn't easy. It's important to offer both compassion towards those struggling and hope that they are not defined by this, it can be overcome.

It's time to choose a different path, one that leads to true healing, not just masked pain. Whether you worry about yourself or a loved one, LEGACY offers a powerful alternative. True healing doesn't just address the physical symptoms of neuropathy – it protects your overall well-being and restores your control over your life.

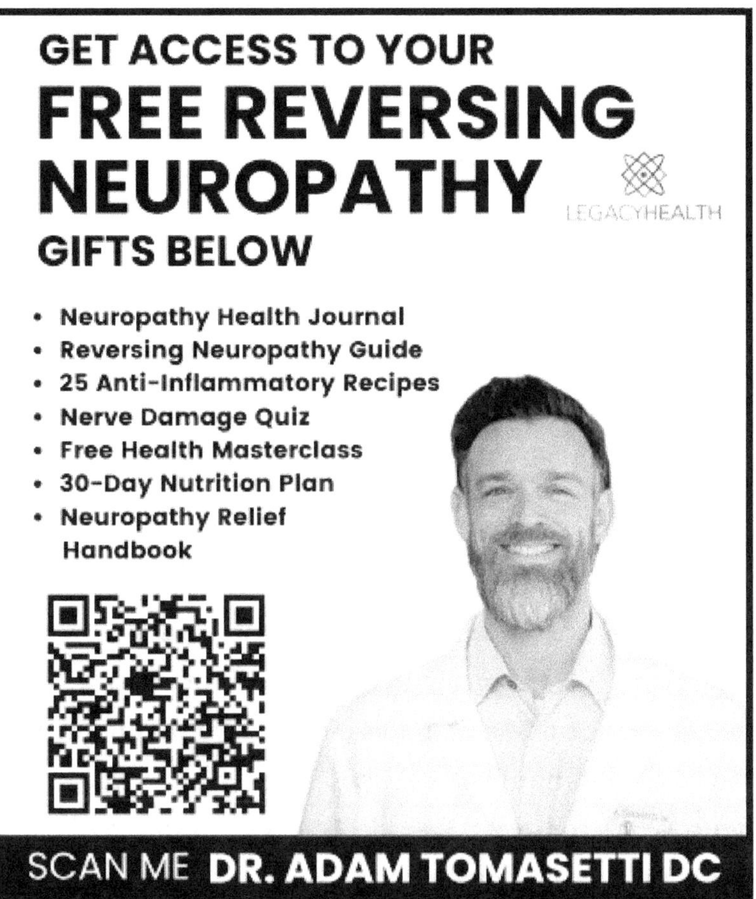

Unlock Your Path to Neuropathy Relief Now: Call 717-285-0001 to Speak With a Skilled Neuropathy Professional Today!

13

THIS IS YOUR MOMENT: BEGIN YOUR L.E.G.A.C.Y. JOURNEY

One of the most rewarding parts of my work is witnessing those moments when the light of hope flickers back on in a patient's eyes. I saw it happen with Mary, a woman in her early 70s who'd been battling neuropathy for over a decade. She'd been told by multiple doctors that she just had to "learn to live with it," and that there was nothing more to be done. She came to me defeated, resigned to a future of limitations and diminishing quality of life.

But Mary had a spark – a refusal to accept this bleak prognosis. She was determined to reclaim her ability to walk on the beach with her grandchildren, to dance at her granddaughter's wedding, to live a life free from the constraints of pain and numbness. That spark is what ignited her commitment to the LEGACY program.

Through a combination of personalized therapies, nutritional guidance, and lifestyle changes, Mary's neuropathy significantly improved. The constant burning in her feet subsided, she regained strength and balance, and most importantly, she rediscovered a sense of joy and possibility that had been missing for years. She was no longer just managing her condition; she was thriving in spite of it.

Disclaimer: Individual results may vary. While many patients experience significant improvement with the LEGACY program, results are not guaranteed. Factors like the severity of neuropathy, individual health history, and commitment to the program all play a role.

Mary's journey is a testament to the power of hope and the transformative potential that exists within each of us. It's a reminder that even when faced with a challenging diagnosis, we have the ability to choose a different path – a path that leads to healing, renewed vitality, and a life lived on our own terms.

Neuropathy has held you back for too long. It's time to break free from its limitations and create a vibrant future for yourself. The LEGACY Neuropathy Program offers a path forward – a path towards healing, renewed hope, and the life you deserve.

The Power of Choice

- **You Can Do This:** The LEGACY Program provides the tools, support, and guidance, but ultimately, your commitment drives success.
- **Change Starts Now:** Everyday you wait is another day neuropathy steals joy. Taking action today initiates positive change.
- **Imagine the Possibilities:** Visualize yourself free from burning pain, sleeping soundly, and walking with ease. This CAN be your reality.

Transformation Is Within Reach

- **More Than Symptom Relief:** The LEGACY approach addresses the root causes of neuropathy, fostering true healing.
- **It's About Quality of Life:** Reclaim the ability to travel, play with loved ones, and participate fully in your passions.
- **You Are Worth the Investment:** An investment in your health is an investment in every aspect of your being.

It's Time to Decide

Are you ready to...

- Commit to a proven, personalized path towards better health?

- Say "yes" to a future where neuropathy has less control?
- Invest in unlocking your full potential for a vibrant, joyful life?

Take Action TODAY

1. **Schedule Your Consultation:** Call Legacy Health (717-285-0001) or visit https://getwellandstaywell.com/health-programs-old/neuropathy-program/ to begin the conversation about your healing. Please note that a consultation is a conversation about your health and does not guarantee specific results. We will work with you to determine if the LEGACY program is right for you and develop a personalized plan based on your individual needs and goals.

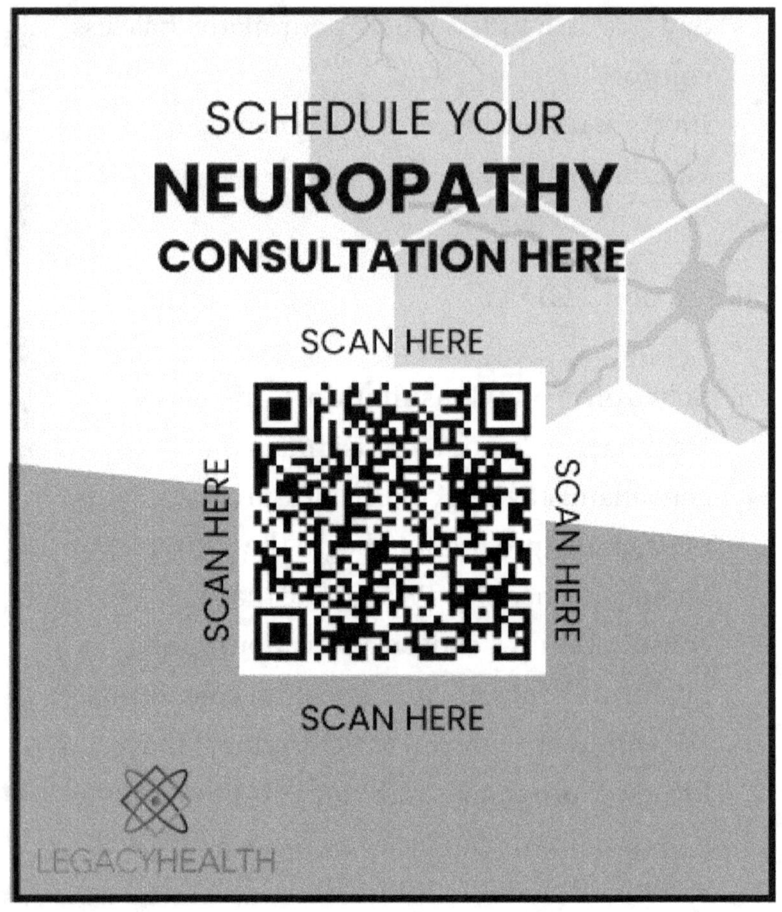

2. **Attend the Informational Workshop:** Text "PAIN FREE" to 717-987-7820 to reserve your seat and get answers to all your questions. This workshop provides valuable information about neuropathy and the LEGACY approach, but does not constitute medical advice or guarantee specific results. It is intended for educational purposes only.

3. **Watch a Free Masterclass:** Not in Camp Hill? Watch our free masterclass to learn more about LEGACY.

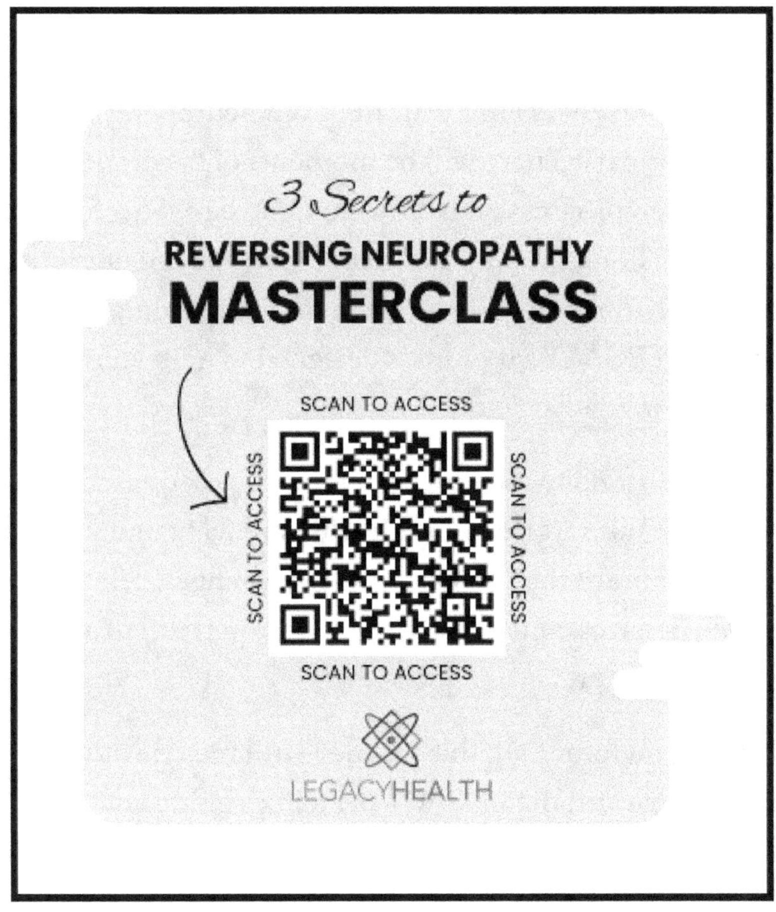

The LEGACY Neuropathy Program isn't a quick fix; it's the start of a transformative process. By taking that first step, you open the door to a better quality of life and a legacy of renewed health and well-being.

As you close this book, I hope you are filled with renewed hope and a renewed sense of control over your health. You've taken a significant step in understanding neuropathy, its impact, and the multitude of ways to find relief.

The journey to reclaim your life from neuropathy won't always be easy. There will be moments of frustration, days when progress feels slow, and maybe even a few setbacks along the way. But remember, you are not alone. Your body possesses an incredible healing power, and the LEGACY Program is designed to help you harness it.

Don't be afraid to advocate for yourself, ask questions, and seek support from your healthcare team and loved ones. Embrace the power of lifestyle changes, celebrate small victories, and never give up on your path to a pain-free future.

Thank you for taking this journey with me. May this knowledge and the LEGACY principles guide you towards a brighter, more vibrant life, where neuropathy no longer holds you back.

With blessings and sincere hope for your healing,

Dr. Adam R. Tomasetti, D.C.